Crisis Intervention in Residential Treatment: The Clinical Innovations of Fritz Redl

Crisis Intervention in Residential Treatment: The Clinical Innovations of Fritz Redl

William C. Morse
Editor

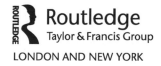

LONDON AND NEW YORK

First published 1991 by The Haworth Press, Inc

2 Park Square, Milton Park, Abingdon, Oxon OX14 4RN
711 Third Avenue, New York, NY 10017, USA

Routledge is an imprint of the Taylor & Francis Group, an informa business

First issued in paperback 2016

Crisis Intervention in Residential Treatment: The Clinical Innovations of Fritz Redl has also been published as *Residential Treatment for Children & Youth, Volume 8, Number 4 1991.*

Copyright © 1991 Taylor & Francis.

Library of Congress Cataloging-in-Publication Data

Crisis intervention in residential treatment : the clinical innovations of Fritz Redl / William´C. Morse, editor.
    p. cm.
    "Also ... published as Residential treatment for children & youth, volume 8, number 4, 1991" — T.p. verso.
    ISBN 978-1-56024-215-4 (hbk)
    ISBN 978-1-138-96697-0 (pbk)
    1. Child psychotherapy — Residential treatment. 2. Crisis intervention. 3. Redl, Fritz — Contributions in child psychotherapy. I. Redl, Fritz. II. Morse, William Charles.
RJ504.5.C75 1991
362.2'1'083 — dc20   91-25834
                                                            CIP

Crisis Intervention in Residential Treatment: The Clinical Innovations of Fritz Redl

CONTENTS

ABOUT THE EDITOR

William C. Morse, PhD, is currently Research Professor at the University of South Florida and Professor Emeritus at the University of Michigan. For many years, he was Director of the University of Michigan Fresh Air Camp, a group therapy camp for disturbed and delinquent boys. The camp also served as a multi-disciplinary graduate training program for pediatricians, psychologists, social workers and teachers of disturbed children. Dr. Morse's recent publications have been on topics such as teaching disturbed children, children at mental health risk, and ecological interventions with disturbed children.

Crisis Intervention in Residential Treatment: The Clinical Innovations of Fritz Redl

Preface

This special edition honoring the contributions of Fritz Redl was conceived by Gordon Northrup, M.D. Gordon Northrup has provided leadership to the cause of residential treatment both by direct service to children and by developing and editing this volume as a channel for professional stimulation to all who are engaged in residential treatment. Like so many of us, he recognized the debt owed to the genius of Fritz Redl and proposed to do something about it.

But Northrup did not propose that we publish a typical eulogy telling new readers what a remarkable man Redl was and what his teachings and leadership meant to our professional careers. Rather, the contributors were to analyze and extend selected contributions of Redl which were applicable to current problems in residential treatment. The highest tribute to Redl is in demonstrating how essential his treatment concepts are for us today, a quarter of a century after the publication of his last collection of papers *When We Deal With Children*.

But there is another purpose to this volume perhaps more poignant. Those who care about the welfare of children in the nineties are being assailed by forces beyond immediate control. There are increasing numbers of children at risk to say nothing of the growing population already seriously disturbed.

Both new and long time workers in the field need the perspective Redl provides as well as his template for day-by-day interaction with very disturbed youngsters. His talent was to challenge the nation's professional leadership and at the same time reach new child care staff: Such was the depth and clarity of his message. If you are concerned about the quality of help disturbed youngsters generally receive nowadays, you want all involved personnel to share Redl's ideas. This is the motivation of the contributors.

There is a saying that accurate insights about child behavior have a life of their own and never die. Insights may not die but they certainly do get lost or covered over. In the vain effort to make child reconstitution easier than it can ever really be, the latest current fad is embraced and the insights of our master teachers neglected. The aim of this volume is to keep the field aware of the treatment truths we learned from Redl so that we do not have to await a subsequent rediscovery and resurrection. Most of all, the children cannot wait: They need this kind of caring right now.

WM

Introduction and Perspective

William C. Morse, PhD

University of Michigan
University of South Florida

These are not the best of times to be a child growing up in the United States. Nor are these encouraging times for professionals concerned about the mental health of youngsters, especially seriously disturbed children and adolescents. Risks escalate while resources shrink. Services are being neglected or reduced in quality. As recent reports from the Children's Defense Fund indicate, reduced resources are taking place in the face of unprecedented threats to the welfare of our children.

Fritz Redl's 1962 presidential address to the American Orthopsychiatric Association was titled "Crisis in the Children's Field." In a later update Redl (1966) wrote that the crisis was still with us, remaining as acute as when he presented his original paper. One wishes we could hear his analysis of the crisis today. He would be speaking out in anger in behalf of our youngsters. The problems Redl described are not only with us still: The fact is the problems are more intense now and they come in new guises. In speaking of the United States and provisions for children, he called us "An Underdeveloped Country, Type II." He explained that a Type II country is one where children's services are sorely undeveloped and for which there is no excuse, this in contrast to traditional undeveloped countries where services of all types are at a primitive state. While we love our kids we neglect our children and virtually hate our youth. He continues his state of the situation address by observing that the available services are flooded with children who do not fit, since they need more than the referral service can provide — should the child be accepted in the first place. Unless there is significant redirection, the 90s will find us continuing as Type II underdeveloped country for children, confronted with an unresolved crisis in child upbringing. It is painful to know that each skirmish won will have to be continually rewon as priorities change with the flux in society.

When one considers the time and energy it takes to produce a healthy youngster in our current society, is it any wonder that re-making a shattered life is financially and psychologically an expensive undertaking? Redl told us that there is no cheap or easy way to provide mental health for children; yet we continue to follow fads and look for short cuts.

Since Redl's work the one significant change in the legal status of seriously emotionally disturbed children has been PL 94-142 passed in 1977. This law delegated to the public schools the responsibility for 'educating' all special children. However well this law has served other categories of special children, it has presented serious problems when it comes to the emotionally disturbed. Why the school and not mental health was given primary responsibility in the first place is an interesting unexplored issue.

At any rate the special education school programs for seriously emotionally disturbed have been recognized as the most problematic and least successful services of special education. The report to the Senate Subcommittee relative to the reauthorization of PL 94-142 which was produced by the National Mental Health and Special Education Coalition (Forness 1989) lists a number of current problems: criterion for identification, training of personnel, liaison with mental health and the delivery of appropriate services among others. Knitzer et al. (1990) examined programs and policies for children with behavioral and emotional problems and concludes there is much wanting in school programs and an overall lack of integrated mental health services for these pupils. She indicates that of the 10 to 30 percent of children in this category needing mental health intervention, less than 1 percent are identified by the schools for special education. Of this under one percent, four percent are eventually placed in residential settings. Overall, she finds over 80% of those identified are educated in the regular public schools (37% in self-contained classrooms) and 12% in day schools or day treatment schools.

In the early days of PL 94-142, much was made of the intended cascade of services, from consultation to the regular classroom teacher, to teacher consultants, resource rooms, special classes (full and part time), day schools and finally full institutionalization. In fact such a cascade of services seldom is available for a pupil. Special classes for the disturbed are being reduced although day schools or day treatment programs are expanding and enroll many of the children who previously would have been institutionalized. The situation is déjà vu to those who saw what happened when adult mental hospitals were emptied out to 'free' the patients to return home to little if any mental health support. Special education is now repeating the process by moving rapidly to what is termed 'inclusion' or mainstreaming. To separate a pupil from normal peers and the normal school setting is perceived as a denial of the child's civil rights. At the same time the many specific services needed to help disturbed children are not being included in the mainstream. To a significant degree only the children who act out or act up (Aldrich 1987) to the point that the system cannot deal with them are placed out and this after a 'significant' event (Barack 1986). Behavior problem children have to exhaust their ecologies first. Depressed and suicidal children are obviously under represented.

Redl's writings and the chapters in this book speak to this current scene in many ways. If more of the children are going to be kept in the mainstream, certainly crisis intervention and Life Space Interviewing are sine qua non. The nature and building of an hygienic milieu assumes importance in all intervention settings for disturbed children, not just in residential placements. Knitzer points out that many school programs are stuck on a point system behavioral modification plateau. The adults have not gone beyond what Redl described as just being able to live in the same environment with disturbed kids. All who work with children need to know more about what makes children "tic," to use Redl's phrase. Aggressive behavior is in long supply but short in our understanding. Delinquency has become endemic. Workers recognize that many disturbed and disturbing children present one self in an individual one to one exchange with an adult and quite another self when performing in a group setting. In our closing section the reader will be directed to certain of Redl's papers on these topics.

The fact is, many young professionals are struggling with difficult children without the advantage of Redl's insights. Those who were long ago introduced to his wisdom will find rereading rewarding for there are always ideas that provide cues for tomorrow's engagements. So let us again become aware of how much we can benefit from his teaching. Fortunately many of the best papers of this remarkable man can be found in his (1966) collection *When We Deal With Children*. The problem is to stimulate directors, professors and students to search out his work and sense the excitement of a writer who was there before we were and writes it like it really is. We can "see" in our experience what he explains in his writings.

No one since has had Redl's clarity of vision combined with the descriptive power to illuminate the meaning of events we live with everyday. His genius was to speak on many levels and present a challenge to the child care worker and theoretician in the same description. The purpose of this publication is to encourage others to find the stimulation Redl's original followers found. Part of Redl's power was in how he delivered the message and unfortunately there is no way this can be reproduced in a printed page even with his colorful turn of phrase. The personality which made such an impact was composed of many facets that touched every writer in this volume as well as thousands who heard him lecture. He was an essential democrat, treating the neophyte and the distinguished with the same warm regard. His sense of humor was always there, and often at his own expense. And Fritz did love a party. He was always in a learning mode. An acute social conscience guided his work. His creativity matched the ease with which he spoke, and his thinking was so organized that there was a logical outline if you took notes. It is no wonder so many have taken him as the model for child mental health professionals.

Unfortunately there is no definitive biography of Fritz Redl, but there is a most fascinating and revealing question and answer discussion by Gottesfeld and Pharis (1977) *Profiles in Social Work*, which Henry Maier pointed out for our benefit, and which should be read in its entirety. The chapter is exciting and informative and will give the reader some of the authentic Redl feeling. Redl crossed more lines than most in his professional career which may account for his open and eclectic approach. He was a teacher in Germany during the period of reformation when less rigid innovations were being tried in schools. For example, once a month a camping trip was required to knit teachers and children through informal activities. His zeal for camping as prime therapeutic environment maintained for life. Also as a teacher he gained his authoritive appreciation of the role of activities in working with children which subsequently contributed so much to his milieu writings. His teaching and camping stimulated his interest in group psychology.

The next phase of Redl's professional development emphasized academic and clinical study. A theoretical depth combined with his hands-on experience made him the stellar expert that he was. In 1925 he earned his PhD from the University of Vienna. There was a close affiliation between analysis and education at that period in Austria: He was trained as a psychoanalyst in the Vienna Psychoanalytic Society. He became a conduit between the analytic founding fathers and later child psychiatry. These experiences were the source of profound theoretical understanding which enabled enlightening interpretations to flow from his keen observations.

The General Education Board brought him to America in 1936 for a study of normal adolescence. When Hitler took over in Europe he stayed, working at the Cranbrook School in Michigan, and then taught simultaneously at the University of Michigan and the University of Chicago as a commuting professor. He became clinical director of the University of Michigan Fresh Air Camp and subsequently organized his own camp, Chief Noonday. These camps embodied both professional training and treatment for disturbed children in a unique action setting. In 1944 came the work with delinquents at Pioneer House in Detroit. Here he emphasized the need for different methods with different types of child disturbance. The concept of marginal interviewing which later became the Life Space Interview was initiated. By this time his 12 year affiliation with the School of Social Work at Wayne University had begun, and he recalled these years as his happiest and most creative period. Again Fritz continued to cross lines between the academic and direct practice which always fertilized his unique creativity. At this time he was much involved with community affairs and what he called clinical group experience.

Redl was a vigorous advocate for children who were suffering in substandard and even corrupt services. His no-nonsense realism and actual experience with difficult delinquents brought him a great following. In 1953 his work moved to NIMH in Washington where he elaborated many of his concepts of treatment for the new type of delinquents. He said delinquents who just needed a well-meaning friendly adult were no more. He worked to help all professionals develop new skills in dealing with these most difficult and socially threatening youngsters. A continuing campaign was his effort to make child care an equal status mental health profession. He often remarked that there was an inverse relationship between the time spent with children and the intensity of professional training. Redl continued to consult in the States and in Europe. He was in contact with the international leaders and continued his writing. The magnetism of the man maintained for the new recruit and the seasoned worker.

Those who have known Redl personally or through his writing want others to have some of the same advantage. Particularly in these times, children need to be served by professionals who espouse what Redl taught and demonstrated. Each contributor to the current volume was given the freedom to select as he or she would, some aspect of Redl's work that had particular pertinence both to the writer and to contemporary mental health care of children. After the long period of 'non-person' behaviorism, the child mental health profession needs to get back to the basics that Redl developed. Some of our contributors worked in direct collaboration with him and indeed made the core of their professional careers from such contact with him. We all knew him for the warm human being he was and for being the most prescient clinician-teacher in our experience. A brief note concerning each contributor follows in order of presentation.

The editor first knew Redl while a student at Michigan while serving as his graduate assistant. He treated me with a democratic respect other professors reserved for their peers. His lectures were lucid and for the first time in the study of psychology I saw how there was a real life counterpart to what was in the books. Students joined him at parties where he was the bon vivant. He introduced a group of us to Christmas in Vienna with St. Nicholas and the Krampus. I knew him as an advocate for children in detention and institutional placement in such reports as *Children Who Rot* and *How to Mangle a Soul*. He was never reluctant to join battle with authorities for the welfare of children. I knew him too as a unique researcher when he directed a milieu study of group behavior at the Fresh Air Camp. Redl was not only my most indelible teacher: He and his wife Helen, became lifelong family friends. Of course I could never follow in his footsteps but, with others of his group, I followed as best I could.

Mary Lee Nicholson has kindly permitted us to print her memorial to Fritz prepared for the service held at Wayne State in 1988. This *Letter to Fritz* catches the spirit of his relationship with colleagues better than could be done any other way. Parallel experiences with Fritz could be repeated for many young professionals. Bandura has pointed out that a life course is usually the consequence of fortuitous events, and here is an example par excellence. If anything is needed to encourage a new generation of Redl readers, her contagious letter should. The pity is there is no possibility of duplicating that experience how: budding new professionals will have to find such inspiration vicariously from his writings as Garfat suggests in a later chapter.

Henry Maier started his association with Redl in 1947 as a counselor in Camp Chief Noonday. Subsequently he served as a fill-in counselor at Pioneer House and started his graduate studies in social work. Wherever he worked from the fifties and on he invited Redl as a consultant or speaker. Also, contacts were maintained at conferences and through solid friendships with a group of co-workers of Redl's projects. "So, over the years I saw him definitely as my 'guru,' teacher, colleague and friend, along with his wife Helen." Maier's paper is a masterful introduction to Redl's work showing how he was ahead of his time in so many ways which is why he is especially pertinent today.

David Wineman was the most involved with Redl of all our contributors. The two were not only colleagues in the School of Social Work at Wayne State University: They were both supervisors and on the line workers at Pioneer House which Fritz directed. The children were the toughest cases collected from Detroit. I can remember vividly Dave and Fritz coming out to the Fresh Air Camp to rescue our staff from the onslaught when this group of kids hit our place. Incidentally, Wineman later became a prime staff clinical leader at that camp where he continued to teach Redl individual and group treatment processes. The classic Pioneer House report on small group treatment homes is found in the joint Redl-Wineman books (1951, 1952) *Children Who Hate* and *Controls From Within*. Wineman's current paper details the way Redl saw the program intertwined with ego support, a major breakthrough in what has become known as ecological intervention.

Nicholas Long has been the most visible extension of Redl both in publication and the conduct of programs. Until recently, while a professor at American University, he directed Rose School in Washington, D.C. This day school and training program was based on Redl's theories. Long began his clinical work at the Fresh Air Camp and was later the director of the school program at the University of Michigan's children's psychiatric inpatient unit. With Wood, he is the author of a new book on Life Space Interviewing (due out in 1991), a skill he teaches at institutes throughout the country. Long's well-known Conflict Cycle extends crisis methodology by providing a paradigm for dealing with aggressive youth. His paper deals with what he learned from Redl about dealing with severely aggressive children, a most appropriate topic if you work in a residence or school these days.

Jerome Beker has written his paper in the tradition of Redl the advocate, lashing out at some of the current stupidity of the mental health profession. In a way, it joins up with Redl's crisis in the children's field mentioned above. Beker's affiliation with Redl was unique, starting when he wrote to Redl as an undergraduate because he wanted to learn more from the man who represented in his writing the kind of a professional Beker aspired to be. Direct contact was at meetings and on editorial boards. Beker is Professor in the Center for Youth Development and Research at the University of Minnesota which he directed for ten years. He crosses lines in Redl fashion, holding appointments in Educational Psychology and the School of Social Work, has an extensive bibliography and is the editor of two child and youth care journals. It is evident that he absorbed Redl's point of view about institutional treatment and therapeutic camping. He argues in his paper that sound treatment follows what the child needs rather than the popular methodological preference of the moment.

The next two papers have to do with Redl and consultation, one as a consultant and the other extending his overall concepts to the practice of consultation. Our first author, Ralph Rabinovitch, has been an innovator in residential treatment, first at the children's psychiatric service at the University of Michigan and later at the outstanding state service he developed at Hawthorn Center, where he invited Redl to consult. Retired from the directorship, Rabinovitch remains active in training and community services for disturbed children. The series of treatment films he produced at

Hawthorn continue to have wide circulation. Always a proponent for the potentials of education in restoring chid mental health, Rabinovitch created the first enriched schooling for seriously disturbed children at the center and pioneered classes for disturbed children in the local public school. He was an advocate for all disturbed and delinquent children and joined with Redl in local action activities. Like Redl, he was always empathic with the plight of parents. One of Rabinovitch's contributions was organizing what soon became a state wide support organization of parents of disturbed children. This association has shown the way parents can monitor and influence state and local mental health programs for children. In his paper, Rabinovitch catches in a delightful manner how Redl worked in a milieu setting to teach both theory and day-to-day child assistance.

Ruth Newman first came to work with Fritz in his NIMH project. As an experienced remedial teacher and clinical psychologist, her job was to organize a school for the aggressive youngsters in the treatment unit. Starting from a state of self-declared naivete she listened and learned and became a professional colleague. Elsewhere she has written a brief paper on what it was like to work with Fritz: a most stimulating, creative and exciting leader, hard to keep up with, spilling out new interpretations and possibilities by the minute. You could depend upon him being there when you needed his support. Her paper introduces us to yet another area of Redl's contributions, and one less well known. Their joint school consultation project harks back to Redl's early professional experiences in teaching and psychoanalysis. There is also a keen awareness of ecological influences found in institutions. As Newman indicates, Redl maintains and extends his dynamic psychology applied here to a new setting but with principles that have a generic application.

The final selection by Garfat harks back to the tribute by Nicholson on what it can mean to a mental health worker to "find" Redl. Since this is no longer possible first hand, Thom Garfat has chosen to dramatize how it still can happen if workers will but sample Redl's writing. Garfat never knew Fritz first hand, or spoke personally with him: only once did he hear him speak. But he tells us that through his writings Redl became a very important influence in his professional life, "it seems that he has always been an integral part of my child and youth care experience." Thom Garfat is the Director of Treatment for Youth Horizons Reception Centre in Montreal, and is co-editor of the Canadian *Journal of Child and Youth Care*. He is a frequent contributor to the field of residential care.

Our recognition of the contribution of Redl closes with an invitation to read Redl. Although Fritz frequently touched on more than one topic in a given paper, certain ones have been grouped to encourage a reader's exploration of given topical areas.

REFERENCES

Aldrich, C.K. (1987). Acting Out and Acting Up: The Superego Lacuna Revisited. *American J. of Orthopsychiatry*, *57*(3) 402-406.

Barack, R.S. (1986). Hospitalization of Emotionally Disturbed Children: Who Gets Hospitalized and Why. *American J. of Orthopsychiatry*, *56*(2) 371-391.

Forness, S. (1989). *Statement of The Mental Health and Special Education Coalition to the Senate Committee on the Handicapped*. Mimeographed, 43 pgs.

Gottesfeld, M.L. & Pharis, M.L. (1977). *Profiles in Social Work*. New York: Human Science Press.

Knitzer, J., Steinberg, Z. & Fleisch, B. (1990). *The School House Door*. New York: Bank Street College of Education.

Redl, F. & Wineman, D. (1951). *Children Who Hate*. New York: Free Press.

Redl, F. & Wineman, D. (1952). *Controls from Within: Techniques for the Treatment of the Aggressive Child*. New York: Free Press.

Redl, F. (1966). *When We Deal With Children*. New York: Free Press.

A Letter to Fritz

Mary Lee Nicholson, MSW

EDITOR'S NOTE: Added to Fritz Redl's professional acumen was a warm, democratic and embracing personality. Thus, those who were privileged to know him were drawn into his circle. Mary Lee Nicholson expresses this most beautifully in this tribute read at Redl's memorial service in Detroit, 1988.

Dear Fritz,

Here is the letter I never wrote to you. I know there will be lots of things said about your magnificent work, your splendid parties, your Pied-Piper capacity to enchant huge crowds of eager listeners.

But, somehow as I sit here on an old Oregon farm, looking out on a spring meadow full of wild daffodils in bloom, I only want to speak of how it was for *me*. I had the incredible luck to cross paths with you at exactly the right time, and I've never been the same since.

In the spring of 1946, I was just finishing a war-time job in Portland, Oregon. I had been out of social work school for two years into the foxholes, long enough to have a few poundings of reality finally make a dent on my delusions of grandeur about work with troubled kids. I had made up my mind never to leave the beauty and freshness of the Pacific Northwest, but the war-time grant that had supported my job ran out, and I was free for the summer.

Just about this same time of the year, I went to a regional conference of the American Camping Association. You were the featured guru. That first evening I almost didn't attend, because an earlier graduate school teacher had haughtily dismissed you one day in class as "that quack in Detroit." Thank God I'm usually impudent enough to take a chance on becoming contaminated by someone

11

without the "proper credentials." Your talk that evening exploded in my head. Here, finally, was someone who MADE SENSE! And you made it with such sparkling, exuberant, right-on-target words and sentences. I had never heard such arrestingly creative combinations before. You, in your second language, were showing me beauty, wit, powerful dilemmas, piercing observations of behavior and its reasons. The Nabokov of professional communication, you were. What a treat. And what a great hope you stirred up in me about what social work *could* be.

Of course you were totally surrounded by an adoring crowd everywhere you went. You were like some partly distracted, friendly Leviathan, moving gracefully along, with a lot of chattering, fawning tug-boats in tow. Someone told you that I might be a person you could interview for a job at Camp Chief Noonday that summer. The interview took place while I sat, cowering, in the back seat of a car driven by an ardent admirer who had kidnapped you for a ride, (just with him, he thought) around the famous seventeen mile drive through the cypress trees along the Pacific. This driver was furious when you insisted that I come along, and he drove ferociously. Meanwhile, you sat turned around in the front seat beside him, serenely conducting a most delightful and totally disorganized interview with me. Neither of us saw a bit of scenery. At the end of that screening ride, I was off to one of the biggest adventures of my life. I went to Michigan that summer, and stayed 18 years.

Few persons are lucky enough to find the right tasks, the right challenges, the right boss, the right colleagues, the RIGHT STYLE, all at the same time. That was your gift to me. You came along just when I needed your unique way of providing the environment where one could struggle, learn, grow, be one's very own self, all in an atmosphere so free, so un-encumbered, so unfraught, so supportive, and so without the usual ego crap that most charismatic persons sooner or later slump into.

You were intrigued with the puzzles, aware of the complexities, full of passionate resistance to *anyone's* bullshit, and able to make those kids very souls come alive for us.

We all eagerly joined you and Dave in your 18 hour days, long, tough weekends, impossible situations, that mocked our best efforts, left us looking and feeling like fools. Yet we kept coming back for more, because you somehow helped it never to be too much, never too daunting, never too crazy. It was magical and exhilarating. We were ok, as long as we all had each other, and the searing needs and mysteries of these kids.

I can see you now, in that old fashioned salt and pepper tweed suit, complete with vest, cigar in hand, nodding that special chin-lifting nod you had for encouragement, chuckling that totally delicious chuckle — unforgettable — at some outrageous happening, being so positively THERE for us that we never felt alone, or out of sync.

Remember the MIDWEST FEELESS FAILURES? We all got so tired of going to conferences where people gave papers on their virtuoso performances, successfully and effortlessly, in twenty pages or less, solving the knotty problems of child treatment. It was always airless in the squalid hotel meeting rooms, we always got charged too much for registration fees, etc. Well, you set a small bunch of us on fire by suggesting that we all get together to discuss only our FAILURES. We took our own food, sleeping bags, slept on each other's floors, met in each other's back yards. That group flourished for several fabulous weekend meetings — in Cleveland, Detroit, Pittsburgh. We all learned profound truths through examining carefully, with your tender help, our biggest work flops.

Fritz, you were such a genuinely GOOD man. You had a sort of gentlemanly, Old World courtliness, almost a remoteness, that sometimes stunned those who pictured you as only the Bon Vivant who banged away on a guitar and sang ribald songs. For me, there was a private, completely non-self presenting side of you that was very comforting. You were a fellow traveller. You could always allow yourself to be the coward who took our cowards' hands. And never, for us, any penalty to pay.

One day, long ago, I came to you in your office in that old rambling house on Kirby before Wayne got so fancy. I was dragging behind me a particularly sticky student problem. I had done all the wrong things. I was ashamed, distraught, self-devouring.

You listened for a long time, looking off in profile as you often did, smoking quietly on the ubiquitous cigar.

On your desk had always been a charming Steuben glass duck — a baby duck — that I had often enjoyed when I was in your office. It was special for you, I know. That day you never said a word in response to my litany of woe, guilt, and perhaps too self-conscious anguish. You picked up that lovely piece of glass, handed it to me gently, and said,

"How about this for *your* desk now, ok?"

What perfection in response — all the layers in tune. That duck still sits on my desk. It's a bit scratched and dulled, but it has soothed and comforted countless over-wrought kids, parents, colleagues, and, always, me, through years of different scenes, different places, different situations.

Goodbye, dear Fritzo. You are missed in so many ways, in so many places. Yet who you were and what you did will reverberate down through all the corridors of time.

The Quakers say it this way —

> Each that we lose
> Yet lives in us
> Our orb grown full and free,
> Draws to itself, at last,
> The tide of immortality.

Bradford Smith, *The Seasoned Mind*

What's Old—Is New:
Fritz Redl's Teaching
Reaches into the Present

Henry W. Maier, PhD

Professor Emeritus
University of Washington

EDITOR'S NOTE: Maier's paper provides an excellent portrayal of Redl's timeliness. We see the introduction of the combined interpersonal and ecological perspectives. With the 'get tough' emphasis today, the exposition on punishment is for all of us. Assessment and treatment were one for Redl. Maier points out that contemporary child and youth care still struggle with Redl's messages.

FRITZ REDL'S WORK:
A PROLOGUE FOR TODAY'S PRACTICE

Redl's innovative ideas of yesterday are very much in evidence and have real relevance for today's child and youth care practices. A truism attributed to Albert E. Trieschman surely applies here as we examine Redl's contributions: "What's old—is new" (Maier, 1988, p. 5).

We find evident, shades of Redl in the current uneasiness with large-scale theories and the replacement of these by situational explorations and practice directions. These ideas were already voiced in the mid-fifties in a little article of Fritz Redl addressed to teachers and mental health practitioners:

Please avoid *any* theories for the time being. This is not the moment to decide just which part of whose stock of knowledge applies best to your case. Your child is still your child, a person of a given age, of given characteristics, who has grown out of very specific circumstances into equally specific character patterns and is doing, right now, very unique and very specific things. You have to look at him [or her] and what he [or she] did long enough to know what is really going on inside and around him [or her]. (1955, p. 4)

This shift, from preoccupation with fitting youngsters into theoretic paradigms toward establishing what is really happening to the youngsters in question and what that behavior then means in the world they and we live in, is essentially in line with today's practice.

Actually, in the 1950s such an admonishment was likewise seen as a paradigm shift; a revolutionary departure from preoccupation with intrapsychic phenomena and with the perception of children's behavior manifested in a vacuum. Redl's *interactional* and *situational* emphases — i.e., understanding children's behavior circumscribed by the world in which they live — are now cited as *interpersonal* and *ecological* perspectives. Today these are established working platforms.

In looking into the work of one of the contemporary leading "gurus," Urie Bronfenbrenner, we find his conceptual framework of ecological human development (1979) akin to Redl's concern with the intervening personal and environmental forces. It is not clear whether Bronfenbrenner actually was familiar with Redl's earlier efforts, but he decisively advanced these earlier concepts.

There seems to be a newly awakened attention to interactive humanistic and ecological factors (earlier identified as "milieu"). They are currently reflected in the human services — especially in group care (Krueger, 1990a). This emphasis is reappearing after decades of experimentation with psychodynamic, behavioral, and other grand-scale formulations for engineering social change.

It is of interest to note that this latest paradigm shift is consistent with events at the end of this century, when political liberalism, an acknowledgment of essential connections across natural and ethnic boundaries as we search for a pluralistic society, is apparently assuming center stage.

Another illustration of the legacy of Redl has to do with his repeated call to perceive "discipline" as an issue of child *care* rather than child control. This was an essential point for him, which he advocated throughout his professional life (1966, pp. 355-377). Especially noteworthy are his strong assaults on physical punishment, which surely had a role in the decline of its use in current child and youth care. Lest we forget this powerful position, his statement and that of Dave Wineman deserves to be cited here:

> We are against the application of physical punishment in any form whatsoever under any circumstances. Even for the normal child we reject the idea that physical pain will "teach" the youngster, that the entrance to the character of a child leads through the epidermis of his hindquarters, or that physical pain will solve things by giving a child the chance to pay for his sins and thus end his guilt feelings. The implication of physical punishment is always, no matter how mild a form is being used, that physical violence will "change" a child, or will motivate him toward a more social approach to life, people, and values. Sometimes it is admittedly meant to be a "behavior stopper" only, but even then we can show the enormous price we pay for such a technique in terms of the poisonous by-products, even should the surface goal be achieved. (1952, p. 211)

In a different sphere of professional concerns it might be of interest for the scope of this publication to note Redl's advocacy to merging child and youth care interests with social work. As early as fifteen years ago, he recommended:

> Right now, I think what should have happened in the field of social work may be a combination of education and the development of child care workers, because as a child care worker you ought to be specially trained; it is a mixture of nursing and social casework and group work. I would like to see child care work as part of social work and nursing combined. (In Gottesfield & Pharis, 1977, p. 91)

Such a merger faltered around 1955; but it was successfully accomplished in the mid-eighties in the University of Pittsburgh's Department of Child Care/Child Development and the School of Social Work. Around the same period, the Center for Research and Youth Development and the School of Social Work came together within one department at the University of Minnesota School of Child and Youth Care; at the University of Victoria, British Columbia, the School of Child and Youth Care and the School of Social Work adopted a mutual commitment to a joint graduate degree program. Thus far, however, these structural unifications have not brought about a substantial merger with educational and practice endeavors.

The major thrust to advance Redl's original pertinent work for the group care field has come from people following his teaching and involved in the training of child and youth care workers. Just to name a few: Jerry Beker (1972, and as editor of the *Child and Youth Care Quarterly*); Larry Brendtro (1969, 1983); Thom Garfat (1985); Mark Krueger (1990a, b); Norman Powell (1990); James Whittaker (1969, 1974); and especially Albert E. Trieschman, by way of numerous well-focused lectures and writings (1969) and the actual practice designs for his residential care and treatment program, the Walker Home and School. Trieschman himself saw much of his practice, teaching, and writing anchored directly in Redl's precepts. It is significant that still today practitioners in the care fields find stimulation and concrete direction for their work in Redl's writings. His contribution to today's group care practice is specifically reflected in the following three areas: (1) assessment and treatment as a multi-faceted experience; (2) from the marginal interview to central care involvement; and (3) teaching as a personal learning experience.

ASSESSMENT AND TREATMENT AS A MULTI-FACETED EXPERIENCE

A report of any single critical event in the life of a child or group of youngsters becomes illuminated by even more questions. These are not merely idle probing questions; for Redl they are exciting moments of search and searching once more (and ultimately research) (1966, p. 17). So much is happening at one time that there can hardly be room for determining exactly whether a response is internal or external, behavioral, affective, or cognitive. The issue whether a behavior is child-or group-centered also fades. Instead, our task becomes to understand children's behavior and to learn what they are expressing rather than under what rubric of classification we should account for their behavior. Redl leaves us breathless in his questioning and excitement over all the possibilities to learn and gain understanding from the children's behavior. It is this enthusiasm about the potential in each assessment that promises an explosion of knowledge and skill attainment. Redl might have equated it to a "scouting" adventure even when looking at so-called routine events. Today, we have become more behavior-specific oriented, as he advocated years ago.

This kind of open-minded assessment leads practitioners away from diagnosis in the more traditional "clinical" sense, which entailed substantiating diagnostic formulations or filling in a grid in the elusive search for causative factors: the *why* of human behavior. Redl was more interested in and found it more useful to look at *how* a behavior occurred. Redl's formulation, emphasizing the circumstances of children's behavior, is coming nowadays to fruition in many residential and kindred care settings where the child no longer stands alone as the subject of scrutiny. It is currently thought that children and youth can best be understood as they are assessed for their interactions amidst their life events. For instance, the event of a girl knocking over her glass of milk has to be studied for the happenings around the table, in the dining room, in her own immediate personal life sphere, as well as her personal dexterity.

In the milk-spilling episode we are concerned about the child's ongoing *experience* rather than her behavior per se. In fact, the designations of a "disruptive child," "misbehaving children," "clumsy" ones, etc., are labels possibly gratifying only to the adults in charge; because they can then exclude themselves and the world around them as agents in the child's misfortune (1975, pp. 569-571). Fritz Redl's perspective found full acceptance in the "revolutionary" '60s and '70s and now in contemporary efforts such as staying away from stereotypically labeling a child as a "mentally retarded child" when actually he or she is a *child* with mental delay. Such a perspective is required to overcome the current questionable practice of describing certain children as "abused children" when actually they are *children* who have experienced abuse and need what every child requires, only more so.

Current-day interest in painstaking efforts to understand the *meaning* of a person's experience or verbal account for its ethnic situational circumstance coincides with Redl's intense exploration into the manifold potential meanings of a single verbal statement. Oliver Wendell Holmes said it succinctly as reported by Jerome Kagan: "A word is not a crystal, transparent and unchanged; it is the skin of a living thought and may vary greatly in color and in content according to the circumstances and the time in which it is used" (Kagan, 1989, p. iii).

Today's disenchantment with digging into a child's past history and scrupulous searching for early childhood trauma are supplemented by the desire to learn more fully the spectrum of the child's or youth's ongoing life experience. This kind of perusal would include the family and beyond; the peers, school, neighborhood, and possibly the community at large (Tracy, 1990). Such a perspective was continuously voiced in Redl lectures and writings. His vivid lectures while on the circuit (always well prepared but frequently merely laid out on the back of an envelope) were full of the myriad of *ingredients* underpinning any one situation.

Nowadays the attention to the specifics, the ingredients of human experience, are also referred to as the "minutiae" of life events (Maier, 1990, pp. 19-20). Fritz Redl once used an example of minutiae: the child who hammered a screw into place. If the youngster had chosen the screw driver, one could infer a different indicator of frustration tolerance. At another time he describes a child interrupting a teacher's talk. He points out the array of possibilities: This child didn't understand, or s/he was eager for gaining teacher or peer good will, or s/he was all excited, anticipating a significant community event coming up, or many other possibilities (1975). All merit significance, because each one gives "the interrupting behavior" its specific tinge. The same dynamics hold for interventive attempts. A caregiver's wink with an eye or a firm hand on a youngster's shoulder can be powerful, minute ingredients to alter an anticipated unwanted behavior of the child.

We are looking here in detail at what Fritz meant with his dictum: "What people really *do* to one another counts as much as how they feel" (1966, p. 86). This concept appears commonly accepted today as a valid psychological, almost a commonsense, perspective. Years back, however, for persons with his psychoanalytic training and his professional alignments, it was a revolutionary pronouncement!

Redl's kaleidoscopic understanding of child and youth behavior requires empathic attention to the impact of environmental (milieu) factors. These include psychological and also *cultural* values (only recently recognized in our actual practice). He would include, as well, factors of which we are just becoming fully aware such as ongoing interpersonal experiences and the controlling and/or allowing aspects of the physical and social settings.

Redl's views are summed up in the succinct subheadings for the first chapter of his and Wineman's *Control from Within* (1952). They interlace all the basic ingredients he felt were paramount for a sound child or youth care environment. These principles, submitted in the fifties, are still, toward the end of the century, true for us but rarely put extensively into operation. A valid care and treatment program requires:

A House That Smiles, Props Which Invite, Space Which Allows
Routines Which Relax
A Program Which Satisfies
Adults Who Protect
Symptom Tolerance Guaranteed, Old Satisfaction Channels Respected
Rich Flow of Tax-free Love and Gratification Grants
Leeway for Regression and Escape
Freedom from Traumatic Handling
Ample Flexibility and Emergency Help
Cultivation of Group Emotional Securities. (1952, p. 11)

Contemporary child and youth care is still struggling with the message of these simple key words, while it is stuck with an earlier fundamental issue: whether care services are essentially control-oriented or life and growth-oriented centers. The orientation previously referred to for maximizing the mental health and personal development of children has yet to find a wide audience in North America.[1]

An additional concern of his had to do with another realm of treatment. In his original style he alerted us to the fact that "We are so much more comfortable with what we are treating children *out of* than what we are supposed to treat them *into*. . . . We give more thought to what kids are like than [we do] what the world we educate and treat them [for] is really like. . . . What the 'reality' in which we want to immerse them actually holds, in terms of health and supportive health ingredients" (1966, p. 31). These poignant concerns are still very much in the wings as we listen to contemporary papers and symposiums in the human service professions.

In the beginning of this decade, emphasis on holistic practice (Powell, 1990), upon contextual and ecological pursuit (Bronfenbrenner, 1979), as well as the recognition of this inherent power derived from each individual and family network (Tracy, 1990; Whittaker, 1979) provide clear traces of Redl's earlier teaching.

Commitment to environmental circumstances brings to mind another Redl twist. It is not merely the impact of the milieu and environmental forces upon the care receivers; also important is what the children do to their environment. A one-dimensional approach becomes multi-dimensional. Child care practice is assuming a new venue. Youngsters in care are seen today, in the words of Lerner and Busch-Rossnagel as "individuals, the producers of their development" (1981). Fritz Redl's challenge is still very much before us in the framework of thinking: What do children do with and to their milieu? In which way can we influence children in our care by assisting them to have an impact on their environments? In other words, can we influence children and youth to discover themselves as partners with their intervening environments? One potential step to accelerate such a progress is reflected in Red's observation that "we have ways [to observe and] to describe *behavior* but not yet the setting and the conditions in which it takes place" (1966, p. 124).

Another departure form the psychoanalytic tenets of his time (a stance well accepted by humanistic-oriented practitioners today) was his focus upon assessing "what is right with the kid." He was interested in what is "right" about the youngsters' skills, peerships, and the opportunities (however undesirable) they may locate for themselves in their home community. He posed the simple technique of establishing what the youngster "*is* doing" in place of what he or she *"is not doing."* The latter merely identifies what the adult thinks a kid should be doing, while the former will bring to light what is actually happening and a fuller account of a child's actual capacities (Maier, 1990, pp. 18-19).

One can only guess at Redl's powerful contribution of *activity engrossment*. This concept surely has had an impact upon our intervention efforts. Fritz Redl's work has centered on the use of play and other activities which engage the child or youth and predictably are apt to join client and worker together; then both the activity and the worker influence the interaction and inherently the treatment efforts.

Control from Within (1952) as well as almost all others of his presentations are filled with the notion of examining activity ingredients which are prone to enhance the flow of the therapeutic experience. In his book (1952) we learn how staff are occupied with finding the "right" program ingredients. Activities like getting up, dressed, making one's bed, etc., are less accounted for, but of course were ever-present in the scheme of things. These were natural, manageable issues tangential to a wholesome experience.

The possibilities for programming kid-centered activities have been advanced in the contemporary scene by such articles as Churchill (1972), Maier (1954; 1985), Pratt (1990), VanderVen (1985), Trieschman and associates (1969), and Whittaker (1974); but basically the potential efficacy of the deliberate use of "program ingredients" has yet to be fully incorporated into basic child and youth care work.

Highlighting the ingredients of therapeutic interaction opens the way to visualizing mental health and child/youth care work as efforts to provide the proper "diets" for individuals. In Redl's terms this would be a "tax-free diet" of basic care. He would clarify that the "diet" mix provided is a prerequisite part of the treatment plan, not to be tampered with, or considered as consequence of good behavior. Such a "diet," to quote Fritz Redl, "has to be guaranteed as an *unbudgetable quantity*. The children must get plenty of love and affection whether they deserve it or not; they must be assured the basic quota of happy recreational experiences whether they seem to 'have it coming' or not. In short, love and affection, as well as the granting of satisfying life situations, cannot be made to be the bargaining tools of educational or even therapeutic motivation, but must be kept tax-free as minimum parts of the youngster's diet, irrespective of the problems of deservedness" (1952, p. 61). Only in the context of such mental health efforts (tax-free) programs will the caregivers have a chance to be seen and experienced as friends rather than masters. Their influence is actualized as the youngsters associate the caregivers with pleasant, strengthening life experiences.

The notion of basic "diets," especially "tax-free" ones, is still much in debate. We could characterize the choice as one of *bestowing* care or of *experiencing* care, conceptualizing the "diet" as an earned privilege or as a fundamental right for each youngster. The "earned privilege" concept is still very much around and in want of Redlism!

FROM THE MARGINAL INTERVIEW TO CENTRAL CARE INVOLVEMENT

We find Fritz Redl's approach most notable in our midst as we review the *role* of residential child and youth care workers of today. His facetious reference to the "psychiatric holy trinity" (psychiatrist, psychologist, and social worker) or his description of interviewing rooms as "pressure chambers" (1966, p. 23) foretold a total reformation to come. Much of the highly guarded interviewing processes are now not merely shared but basically taken over by the care workers in residential settings. It is they who are the ones in the frontline of care, who share in the youngsters' daily life experiences.

"Marginal interviewing," coined by Redl and Wineman (Redl, 1959b; Wineman, 1959) hints at a too wide marginality in the "therapeutic interview" set at a fixed time and place with a special set of professionals; it advocates being marginally near or as *close* to the incident as possible. It encourages dealing with the happening while it is *hot*, at the scene of action. (In Redl's colorful phrasing: "therapy on the hoof.") A therapeutic exploration, they submitted, should be done by those on hand at the moment. One outcome of this approach has been the recognition of the meaningfulness of such encounters, and this has led to frontline workers assuming basic counseling functions, becoming essential treatment agents during the children's and youths' placement; they become involved in liaison work with the youngsters' families and eventually, at a number of residential programs, also attend to actual family work (Garfat, 1990; McElroy, 1988). Undoubtedly, with care workers assuming instrumental therapeutic treatment functions in these so-called "life-space" encounters, we have now come to see these workers as vital treatment partners, as members of *the team*.

Also, the Redl and Wineman emphasis on marginal or life-space interviews has lured members of the "trinity" themselves to become involved at times in the residents' day-to-day group life. Visiting the units, joining in meals or play periods and other casual interactions in the youngsters' own life space has provided opportunities for important contacts with their clients.

Life-space interviews have, in essence, moved counseling or therapeutic work to a stance of mediation between the child and what life holds for him or her (1966, p. 37). Currently, this concept is well designated by Thom Garfat as "counseling on-the-go" (Garfat, 1985); that is, counseling occurring closest to the experience, shared by the person most involved at that moment. We can sense in this assertion the slogan of the sixties: "here and now!" While Redl viewed life-space as an experiment, a potential vital avenue for direct involvement in a child's or youth's experience (1966, pp. 35-67), today this idea has blossomed into many avenues of human services.

The idea and actual practice to work as close as possible to the scenes of relevant daily life of the individuals concerned have been translated into work in the streets, at daycare, school, and playground or fast-food places, and particularly in their homes. Especially noteworthy is the emerging service of child development care workers in elementary schools (trained social workers in the U.S. and child care workers in Canada), as well as genuine family work offered within the family's own quarters (Garfat, 1990). Such programs are typified by Homebuilders (Kinney et al., 1990), where the thrust is to deal with the issues of family maintenance and change whatever the immediate tasks might be. In short, the once modestly designated "marginal work" is more and more emerging as *central* to treatment efforts. And the once traditional in-office

interview hour has given way to short and extended life-space en-
tanglements. Al Trieschman and associates' classic *The Other 23
Hours* (1969) could now be plagiarized as "23 Hours and the Other
One"!

TEACHING AS A PERSONAL LEARNING EXPERIENCE

In the foregoing pages, Fritz Redl's techniques have been reviewed for their far-reaching effects into the contemporary practice.
So much of his material has found an audience, and more significant, a way into contemporary practice approaches. After all, when
Redl spoke, people listened! One wonders if his unique *teaching
skills* have transferred into present-day efforts as well. His style of
communication really conveyed his message.

Shades of this master teacher are in evidence today when trainers
emulate his delivery by investing a heavy dose of personal energy
into the material presented. This investment represents an effective
way to convey the presenter's personal conviction about the material to be learned.

Today's acceptance of an a-theoretical approach to human behavior and development—bordering on eclecticism—might be directly
traced to Redl's breaking away from a single point of view and
eagerly incorporating other sources of knowledge regardless of their
divergent bases. Teachers who are open learners themselves, we
observe, are the effective teachers.

Youth and child care conferences and publications of the present
day seem to be characterized by their lively illustrations and presentations of critical incidents relating to the presenters' teaching
points. Surely these efforts are in tune, at the very least, with Redl's
former lectures, full of rich anecdotes and colorful illustrations,
bringing the reader or listener right there as a learning participant.
Interesting, too, is the observation that teachers in the social and
human sciences currently focus on situational rather than case history circumstances. Fritz, a man ahead of his time, also diverged
from case histories, as evidenced in all of his publications.

There are two other facets of his teaching which should perhaps
be acknowledged, although these may not have fully percolated into
the present scene: He made continuous efforts to explore alternative

interventions. His teaching reflected a constant search for added bits of wisdom. He hardly ever was content with any *one* overriding answer. He thought that each situation could yield multiple answers, and he instilled in his readers and listeners the desire to explore what can become knowable.

In a similar vein, he was attracted to life's dilemmas and interactions which do not proceed as anticipated. In short, he was drawn to practitioners' frustrations and their professional "failures" as practitioners. *In Controls From Within* (1952), he alluded with dignity to the rich learning and added insight he, Wineman, and staff acquired from their "mistakes." In her moving farewell to Fritz Redl, Mary Lee Nicholson (in this issue) cites the genuine excitement she and her associates experienced as they reviewed and explored with him the "failures" in their work. This validates the notion that learners are the explorers of new territories; they don't profit so much from proving what they already know as they do from delving into what needs to be understood more fully. Here in our training or counseling we have not yet found ways to utilize failures as springboards for subsequently effective learning.

CONCLUDING OBSERVATIONS

Undoubtedly, we have experienced a paradigm shift in recent years in child and youth group care, and in particular in the residential care and treatment fields. It has been marked by a shift from a general preoccupation with the youngsters' psychic life development to a pronounced attention to their ongoing life-styles and circumstances, with a search for opportunities for change within their particular life spheres. Redl served as both a proponent and deliverer of such change. He stands tall both in finding a "tolerance toward the meaning of old ideas" (Kagan, p. 67) and in alerting his students to new perspectives which, toward the end of this century, have become in many ways a foundation for ongoing practices.

And finally, it might be apropos to fall back upon two astute observations of Redl's, one from the earlier days of his professional career and the other as a voice within the last decade, toward the end of his career, with profound impact. First, the more recent one: In 1982, in a taped interview, he reminded us that our mutual struggle for *basic* acceptance of children, thereby achieving effective care work with and for children, is still somewhat unfulfilled. "Now we have to go back and convince people they have to care about their children. . . . Usually the Bible, a legend or so, a societal taken-for-grantedness took care of it. Now we discovered we have got to convince people. . . . That's pretty frightening" (Redl, 1982).

Lastly, in one of his earlier writings, ten years after resettling in the United States, he noted that in times of emergency and strain we are apt to get all excited about the problems we have not solved, and to tend to forget the things which have been achieved. This, he said, is not a singular lack of forward-mindedness. The difficulties are likely more related to the fact that new effective approaches are masked by old arrangements and structural hangovers (1944, p. 16).

We find Fritz Redl's concerns for children, youth, and their caregivers reaching well into the present. Or, as Al Trieschman described it, Fritz continues to be "a twinkle in the eyes" for the present generation in the child and youth care fields.

NOTE

1. It is important to note that Redl's contributions are effectively applied, among others, at such care centers as the Walker Home and School and Cottage V of the William Roper Hull Institute. These selected places, for instance, do not depend on any form of fancy "therapeutic hour" but what has an impact on the residents throughout their many hours and days in group care.

REFERENCES

Beker, J. (1972). *Critical incidents in child care*. New York: Behavioral Publications.

Brendtro, L. K., Ness, A. E., & Milburn, J. F. (1983). Psychoeducational management: Individualizing treatment. In L. K. Brendtro and A. E. Ness (Eds.), *Troubled youth: environment for teaching and treatment* (pp. 127-133). New York: Aldine Publications.

Bronfenbrenner, U. (1979). *The ecology of human development*. Cambridge, MA: Harvard University Press.

Churchill, S. R. (1972). Pre-structuring group content. In J. K. Whittaker and

A. E. Trieschman (Eds.), *Children away from home* (pp. 311-320). New York: Aldine.

Garfat, T. (1985). *Reflections on the words of Dr. Fritz Redl.* Montreal, Que.: Youth Horizons. Unpublished paper presented at the First International Child and Youth Care Conference, Vancouver, B.C.

Garfat, T. (1990). The involvement of family as consumers in treatment programs for troubled youth. In M. A. Krueger and N. W. Powell (Eds.), *Choice in caring* (pp. 105-143). Washington, D.C.: Child Welfare League of America.

Gottesfield, M. J., & Pharis, M. E. (1977). Fritz Redl. In *Profiles in Social Work* (pp. 73-94). New York: Human Science Press.

Kagan, J. (1989). *Unstable ideas, temperament, and self.* Cambridge, MA: Harvard University Press.

Kinney, J., Haapala, D., Booth, C., & Leavitt, S. (1988).The Homebuilders model. In J. K. Whittaker, J. Kinney, E. M. Tracy, & C. Booth (Eds.), *Improving practice technology for work with high-risk families: Lessons from the "Homebuilders" social work education program.* University of Washington, School of Social Work, Center for Social Welfare Research, Seattle, WA (Monograph #6), pp. 37-68.

Krueger, M. A. (1990a). Child and youth organizations. In M. A. Krueger & N. W. Powell (Eds.), *Choice in caring* (pp. 1-18). Washington, D.C.: Child Welfare League of America.

Krueger, M. A. (1990b). Principles and themes in child and youth care work. Unpublished manuscript, University of Wisconsin, Outreach Department, Milwaukee, WI.

Lerner, R. M., & Busch-Rossnagel, N. A. (Eds.). (1981). *Individuals as producers of their development: A life-span perspective.* New York: Academic Press.

Maier, H. W. (1987). *Developmental group care of children and youth.* New York: The Haworth Press, Inc.

Maier, H. W. (1988). Foreword. In R. W. Small & F. J. Alwon (Eds.), *Challenging the limits of care* (pp. 5-9). Needham, MA: The Walker Home and School.

Maier, H. W. (1985). Essential components in care and treatment environments of children and youth. In *Development group care of children and youth* (pp.19-70). New York: The Haworth Press, Inc.

Maier, H. W. (1990). A developmental perspective in child and youth care work. In J. P. Anglin, C. J. Denholm, R. J. Ferguson, & A. R. Pence (Eds.), *Perspectives in professional child and youth care* (pp. 7-24). New York: The Haworth Press, Inc.

Maier, H. W., & Loomis, E. A. (1954). Effecting impulse control in children through group therapy. *International Journal of Group Psychotherapy, 4,* 312-320.

McElroy, J. R., Jr. (1988). The primary caretaker model: A developmental model for the milieu of children and adolescents.'' In R. W. Small & F. J. Alwon (Eds.), *Challenging the limits of care* (pp. 29-43). Needham, MA: The Walker Home and School.

Powell, N. W. (1990). The conflict cycle: A useful model for child and youth care workers. In M. A. Krueger and N. W. Powell (Eds.), *Choice in caring* (pp. 19-38). Washington, DC: Child Welfare League of America.

Pratt, S. (1990). Therapeutic programming and activities: Transitional tools in the treatment process. In J. P. Anglin, C. J. Denholm, R. V. Ferguson, and A. R. Pence (Eds.), *Perspectives in professional child and youth care* (pp. 59-70). New York: The Haworth Press, Inc.

Redl, F., & Wineman, D. (1951). *Children who hate*. Glencoe, IL: The Free Press.

Redl, F., & Wineman, D.(1952). *Controls from within*. Glencoe, IL: The Free Press.

Redl, F. (1955, December). Who is delinquent? *National Parent Teacher*.

Redl, F. (1959a). The concept of a therapeutic milieu. *American Journal of Orthopsychiatry, 29,* 721-730.

Redl, F. (1959b). Strategy and technique of the life-space interview. *American Journal of Orthopsychiatry, 29,* 1-18.

Redl, F. (1966). *When we deal with children*. New York: The Free Press.

Redl, F. (1975). Disruptive behavior in the classroom. *School Review, 83,* 561-594.

Redl, F. (1982). Quoted from videotape. In M. A. Krueger, *Principles and themes in child and youth care work*. Unpublished manuscript, University of Wisconsin, Outreach Division, Milwaukee, WI.

Redl, F., & Sheshiakov, G. V. (1944). *Discipline* (pp. 16-65). Washington, DC: National Education Association.

Tracy, E. M. (1990). Identifying social support resources of at-risk families. *Social Work, 35,* 252-258.

Trieschman, A. E., Whittaker, J. K., & Brendtro, L. K. (1969). *The other 23 hours*. Chicago, Aldine.

VanderVen, K. (1985). Activity programming: Its development and therapeutic role in group care. In L. C. Fulcher & F. Ainsworth (Eds.), *Group care practice* (pp. 155-186). New York: Tavistock.

Whittaker, J. K. (1974). Program activities: Their selection and use in a therapeutic milieu. In P. Glasser, R. C. Sarri, & R. D. Vinter (Eds.), *Individual change through small groups* (pp. 237-250). New York: The Free Press.

Whittaker, J. K. (1979). Developing community linkages. In *Caring for troubled children* (pp. 124-136). San Francisco: Jossey-Bass.

Wineman, D. (1959). The life-space interview. *Social Work, 4,* 3-17.

Fritz Redl:
Matchmaker to Child and Environment —
A Retrospective

David Wineman, MSW

Professor Emeritus of Social Work
Wayne State University

EDITOR'S NOTE: After clarifying Redl's unique talent in diagnostic use of observation, Wineman's paper elucidates Redl's contribution to understanding ego breakdown in delinquent and aggressive behavior. He continues with discussion of antiseptic handling of such behavior, including life space interviewing and milieu design.

Dr. Norman Polansky once described Fritz Redl as a "genius at pulling significant behavior out of the raw mass," referring to Redl's phenomenal skill at recognition and description of diagnostically critical individual behavior. Redl's writings reveal an equally remarkable talent at envisioning and assessing *environmental* structures and processes for their impact on children's needs, coping abilities and implications for growth and maturity. His major professional and intellectual contribution to the children's field springs from his creative use of these two gifts in his conceptualizations of "total treatment design" for the ego-disorganized, aggressive child.[1] In what follows I attempt to give a nuts and bolts (if only bird's eye) view of this extraordinary feat of visionary thought and action in bringing child and environment together. Also, some brief comments are included regarding the significance of Redl's work in the changing psychoanalytic thought of the mid-20th century and his challenge to do behavioral research.

EGO BREAKDOWN ON THE SCENE
OF DAILY LIFE

Redl's description of ego disorganization in the aggression-filled young delinquent is concrete and empirical. In *Children Who Hate* (Redl & Wineman 1951) some 23 commonly occurring mini-collapses of ego functioning in the children's daily lives are documented, criss-crossing major areas of the control system. For example, fear and anxiety from any source, however mild, often result in complete breakdown of controls, precipitating total flight and avoidance, or ferocious attack and diffuse destructiveness. Similar failures occur in dealing with mistakes, disappointments, case history flare-ups, coping with even mild temptation, or with unexpected gratification, and even with success or victory in a game. And, while more normal youngsters tend to use materials in ways that are consistent with their inherent potential to offer gratifications, these children show a kind of "sublimation deafness" tending to use objects and materials to gratify basic urges directly. Redl argues that the breakdown and disorganization of ego-adaptive functions on the daily life scene is itself a causal source of hate from the pure overflow of stress and frustration thereby engendered. This system of hate is also seen, however, as being fed by developmental trauma and past nurturance deficits, in this way reflecting traditional theory's claims of the damages of libidinal neglect.

As though the stored-up inner misery of such children and the poverty of their coping functions do not present an enormous enough clinical challenge, still another fascinating but tortuously baffling complexity stares us in the face. Side by side, with the puniness of the children's ego functions, there lies an enigmatic and unexpected power. The selfsame ego, so unable to cope with the impulses themselves and other minimal daily stresses, suddenly, with an exasperating and ruthless efficiency, performs super-human tasks in defending impulse gratification at all costs rather than showing any tendency to reconcile reality demands, desires and social values.

This "delinquent ego" is depicted as battling on four fronts against surrender of impulse gratification: (1) by the ingenious use of *defenses against inner guilt, embarrassment or shame* that could result from whatever rudiments of superego that might reside in the inner self; (2) by alertness and tirelessness in *searching for delinquency* support, both externally (such as in expert "diagnosis" of and immediate alliance with other delinquents, or in refusal to budge from delinquency supportive environments), or internally, from within the self (such as "You know what a lousy temper I've got — how could I help clobbering the son-of-a bitch!?''); (3) by *direct defense against change* when exposed to situations which present a frontal exposure of the delinquent side of the self (such as not being able to admit a theft in the face of unshakable evidence and total immunity from punishment), and (4) through *"mechanized warfare against change agents,"* involving such techniques as attempts to weaken staff morale through "anticipatory provocation" — efforts to lure adults into mean, hostile rejecting behavior — or an amazing range of highly fluent, sophisticated legalistic arguments as counter-interview techniques when it came to an attempt to lure them into a confession of a misdeed or confront them with a particularly untenable piece of behavior, or to shock them into an admission of guilt, unfairness or what not, related to a specific incident in their group.

This describes another major target at which the treatment design must take aim, and which exponentially increases the complexity of the strategic and tactical issues at hand. For, these children for whom adult affection is virtually a life giving necessity, fear it as much as they need it. They are caught in the dilemma of dammed if they do and damned if they don't. If they accept gratification and love, their intuitive fear, despite all their ego confusion, is that their license to impulse freedom is in jeopardy. If they don't, and continue to exercise their awesome ability to serve their illicit impulse gratification master, they fear they may jeopardize the new "gratification package" at the source.

"On the ground," especially in the beginning, the children deal with this by greedily gobbling up everything given while at the same time waging holy war against the givers!

TOTAL TREATMENT DESIGN

Redl's paradigm of the ego dysfunctional, impulse ridden child presents the prima facie case for his contention that only a total treatment design in which every phase of the residential setting is involved could confront the full range of clinical challenges presented.

His writings on total design reveal both his passion for achieving a *best-fit* in the child-environment system and his genius at visualizing what might be called *the psychosocial composition of clinical life space* or *regions* which would conform to this criterion. His blueprint is a composite of three distinct and overlapping regions in which children and staff reciprocally interact over time and are tied to the three major treatment need patterns of the children: (1) recuperation from the traumatic, primitivizing and anti-nurturant past via "tax free love" and gratification "grants," (2) access to an intricate and varied network of daily supports and activities which address needed adult-child relationship processes, allow hygienic behavioral control, and provide structured ways for adding new functions and skills to ego adaptive repertories, and (3) overcoming "delinquent ego" warfare against treatment acceptance and change.

REGION 1

Antiseptic Handling of Surface Behavior

The residential clinician who directly lives with the surface behavior of the children constantly faces behavior requiring instant interference for reality reasons totally disconnected from any therapeutic goal.[2] A ferocious physical attack by one child on another, or a child over-stimulated by group excitement and on the verge of disastrous behavior, or a sadistic scapegoating episode, do not raise the case history issues of *why do these youngsters need to do these things* or *what has led up to their basic disturbances*. The issue is strictly and clearly the stopping of one brand of behavior or the production of another.

But, while the clinically-oriented intervenor in child behavior wants something that really works to cut the sadistic teasing or quickly remove the over-excited kid who throws the first piece of watermelon in the dining room before he sets off a contagion chain, he will be equally concerned that what is being done *is at least harmless in terms of its side effects on the basic clinical goal*. Beyond this, Redl also insists that the right type of interference strategically applied is sometimes the very thing that constitutes an important step in a direct therapeutic task.

Redl describes seventeen distinct varieties of interference ranging from "planned ignoring" to "physical restraint." Each is examined in relation to a prototype of behavior — sometimes whole behavioral scenes — for which it is best suited transactionally, by which I mean would create the best fit between what the kid is experiencing and what the intervenor would do (as judged by the twin test of effectiveness and antisepsis.) The phenomenological thoroughness with which these are examined, the attention to the ego and superego dynamics of behavioral control and the care with which pro and con analysis is carried out, do in fact appear to put Redl's categories of antiseptic management somewhere *between* behavioral stoppage and clinical maneuvering. Consider this typical example from only a portion of an analysis of what he terms "Signal Interference" to catch the flavor of proximity to a clinical process (Redl and Wineman 1952):

> A great deal of wild behavior occurs not because a child has no judgment about the danger implied or no value sensitivity about its unacceptability but because his ego or superego doesn't happen to be vigilant enough at the moment to prevent it or has been waylaid or swept aside by a momentary upsurge of seductional challenge. There is a difference, of course, between the youngster who is engaged in a feud against a neighbor whom he has placed in the category of an enemy and about the destruction of whose property he has from now on not the slightest compunction and the youngster who is fascinated by the temptation of climbing which the neighbor's cherished hedge may temporarily throw into his path. In the first case, it would be silly to expect him to drop his destructive escapade by any but rather direct and heavy means of interference. In the second case, it may be sufficient to signal to the otherwise vigilant ego or superego of the child which from then on takes

over and suppresses the seductive impulse which was just about ready to emerge. Thus, a youngster who is suddenly fascinated by the challenge of hurdling the neighbor's hedge will easily respond if the counselor to whom he is well related and who caught the sudden gleam in his eye makes some clear gestures of disapproval, like waving his finger, or saying "uh uh," or whatever the customary signal is. Of course, a group of youngsters who are ready to burst into a riotous breakdown of overexcitement around the dinner table will not stop throwing food or knives unless they are actually held or strongly interfered with. If, however, the gradual trend in the direction of that mischief is discovered earlier, at a time when the youngsters are still adult-related and when their original group code about behaving a little more reasonably around the dinner table is still basically intact, it may again be enough for the adult to give a clear signal of unacceptability of that behavior in a friendly way. This signalling of the unacceptability of the behavior will block the rising disorganization. (pp. 160-161)

REGION 2

Activity Programming as a Therapeutic Tool

Few, if any, in the field of residential treatment of children rival Redl's intense absorption with the designing of activity programming as a full-fledged therapeutic tool, based upon his conception of the psychodynamic impact of activity on the impulse control balance of the child.

His thesis basically is as follows: children in general, and especially deprived, hostile, gratification hungry children, often appraise the amount of affection or rejection they receive from adults primarily through activity channels. Further, and again, especially with the impulse driven child (even assuming the most heroic performance of antiseptic intervention!), the unavoidable frequency of interference by adults or of situations which are frustrating to the children cuts down on the amount of love signals which adults can give. The most friendly and affectionate adult is perceived by them in many moments of the day as a hostile, negative interferer and even as an enemy. A treatment home, therefore, especially in the beginning, has to rely heavily on indirect channels of communication of acceptance and affection from adults. One of the safest indirect channels is the amount of gratification the children receive during a day *and the willingness and enjoyment on the side of the adult* with whom they are allowed to receive it. Indeed, children may engage in the happiest recreational experiences but, if they think that the adults frown upon them, they interpret these experiences not as a symbol of love from adults, but as a triumphant prize won against their vigilance. It is, therefore, important that the institution as a whole and every person in it are openly and explicitly acceptant of children having "fun."

But, since Redl approaches program as a full-fledged therapeutic tool dedicated not only to fun but ego support and repair, the goals of raising the children's acceptance level of higher demands of impulse organization and ability to gain pleasure from more sublimated outlets of their impulses are important to pursue. The following citation from a much longer discussion by Redl of this issue illustrates the complexity and theoretical liveliness with which he treats this question, as well as such activity related variables as frustration avoidance and "budgeting," concessions to children's sociological taste patterns and past "fun habitats," individual antisepsis, group psychological hygiene, protective timing, program "hangover" effects, uses of positive interest contagion, among still others (Redl and Wineman 1952):

> The "level of organization" to which we could subject our youngsters at different times, as well as the "primitivity of gratification" we had to yield to, or the "sublimation demands" we could make under favorable circumstances, would vary greatly. The real problem the practitioner faces in connection with this item is simple to state: We usually consider higher organization levels, as well as less primitive and more sublimated gratification channels, more desirable and educationally "valuable." The trouble is, are they still fun? And while we can lure some children some of the time into concessions on this point, one of our tasks is not only to get them to concede to us their participation in activities which demand higher organization and higher sublimation levels, but to get to the point where they can even enjoy them. The educator usu-

ally hopes to move them to "higher levels" on both counts. The clinician wants to be sure he knows just how much organization and sublimation they can really take without their ego being loaded with an unbearable weight of frustration or anxiety. The clinician, then, would make two demands on program planning: one, that it be "realistic," so that it will expose youngsters to activity levels which they can enjoy without having to expose their ego to a breakdown, and, two, that it be "challenging" in the long run, which implies making provisions that the ego gets enough support, so that it occasionally can cope with higher organization and sublimation demands than it otherwise could. (pp. 106)

REGION 3

The Life Space Interview

Quite often the child with severe coping disturbances needs more than the on-the-spot tactics referred to in discussion of "antiseptic intervention" to "make it" in group situations with other children and adults. Behavioral situations arising from within or without (or both) may require emergency help of interview proportions conducted in close proximity to the actual scene in which the behavior erupted, but at the side of the "action," or close by in a convenient room or corner. After some years of experience with these occurrences, for which Redl coined the term "life space interview," he differentiated two basic functions that were being served. In one which he called "emotional-first-aid-on-the-spot" the objective is short range and present oriented: re-establishment of ego control sufficient to get the youngster back into the program, a kind of elongated and more complex "antisepsis." The other, termed by Redl "clinical exploitation of life events," is long range and future oriented and attempts to extract from the experience involved whatever clinical gain might be drawn from it for long range treatment goals.

Redl argues that the strategically wise use and technically correct handling of life space interviews are of foremost clinical importance and involve as important issues of strategy and technique as do decisions the clinical practitioner has to make during the therapeutic hour (Redl 1966; Wineman 1959).

While space limitation allows mainly their labels, the following chart of life space interview sub-functions may serve to indicate their wide tactical scope, from ego support to ego repair, in addressing ego-environment issues, internal blockages in the freeing of pre-conscious value sensitivities, personal autonomy and symptom denial.

Emotional 1st Aid

1. Draining off frustration "acidity"

2. Providing support in moments of panic, fury and guilt

3. Maintaining communication in moments of "relationship decay"

4. "Umpire" services (between kids and in individual decision-making crises)

5. Regulations of behavioral and social traffic ("traffic cop" function; strategic reminders of basic ground rules)

Clinical Exploitation

1. *Reality "Rub-In":* Magnifying dimly perceived reality events; confronting paranoid-like "life interpretations"

2. *Sympton Estrangement:* Decreasing symptom comfort and secondary gain

3. *"Massaging" numb value areas:* value repair and restoration; increasing ego tolerance for guilt-tension

4. *New tool "salesmanship":* providing new coping skills in moments of problem solving challenge

5. *Manipulation of boundaries of the self:* increasing ego autonomy in face of group excitement, group psychological "suction," and temptational "lure"

"Just How Does the Milieu Do It?"

Clearly, while retaining the Freudian structural model Redl sees its constituent functions and processes as an *open system*, freely interacting with the surrounding environment. His approach — holistic, multifocal, present oriented — swings radically away from the atomistic, past-oriented, reductionism of the classical model.

But if ego psychology with its emphasis on ego autonomy and adaptive functions, provides a partial, conceptual framework for Redl's milieu theory, it tells us nothing about what happens once the action begins. The blueprint with its enormous success at visualization of finely-honed missiles to hurl at pieces of ego and superego dysfunction, and libidinal wreckage from the past, is one thing. But, "Just how does the milieu do it?", Redl asks in a provocative paper on the therapeutic milieu. In answer he urges highly focused research observation and tracking of specific ingredients, making it clear that children are never hit by the milieu as such but always in a specific form and at a given time and place (Redl 1966):

> Rather than studying the "milieu" per se and then the "reactions of the children," how about making it a four-step plan? Let's keep the "milieu" as the over-all concept on the fringe; its basic ingredients come close to my youngsters only insofar as they are contained in a given setting. For example, my children on the ward can be found engaged in getting up and eating meals or snacks. They can be found roaming around the playroom or in a station wagon, with all their overnight gear, on the way to their camping site. They can be found in their arts-and-crafts room or schoolroom engaged in very specific activities. Enough of illustrations. The point is in all those settings the whole assortment of milieu aspects hits them in very specific forms: There is an outspoken behavioral expectation floating through the arts-and-crafts room at any time. There are spatial characteristics, tools, and props. There is the potential reaction of the other child or adult, the feeling tone of the group toward the whole situation as such; there is the impact of people's goal values and attitudes, as well as that of the behavior of a child's neighbor who clobbers him right now

with his newly made Viking sword. In short, I may be able to isolate observations of milieu ingredients as they "hit" the child in a specific setting during a specific activity. On such a narrowed-down level of observation, I may also be able to trace the actual experience that such a concrete situation in a given setting produced in the child; and if I know what the child did with the experience, it may make sense, for I have both ends of the line before me: the youngster's reaction to his experience and the nature of the ingredients of the "setting" on both ends of the line, plus plenty of good hunches on the child's experience while exposed to its impact. (pp. 92-93)

This is the voice of Redl as believer in a full measure of naturalistic observation as the first step in trying to understand causality. As a research thinker Redl was less than happy with modern behavioral researchers' fixation on quantification, control machinery and "neatness in hypethesizing" before they really knew what they should be looking at. "Let's put the search back into research," he pleads in a seminal paper, based on his 1961 presidential address to the American Association of Orthopsychiatry. Redl's challenge to behavioral research remains unanswered.

Few of those in the children's field could think like Fritz Redl about the lives of children. He was always fresh, always in perfect rapport with their world whether in an action setting with live kids — camp, treatment home, ward — or lecturing to a seminar of ten or to a thousand psychiatrists at an Orthopsychiatry conference. He was a magisterial illuminist, emitter of a never-ending cascade of brilliant ideas in delightful, exciting and comprehensible forms that painlessly conveyed theoretical complexity and depth. He had wit, warmth, and optimism. The legacy of his wisdom, a movable feast, is a precious source of nurturance for the minds and spirits of all, from the playground to the consulting room, who "deal with children."

NOTES

1. Quotes throughout refer to terms Redl originated or typical language he would use.

2. For a more detailed discussion see Redl and Wineman, 1952.

REFERENCES

Redl, F. & Wineman, D. (1951) *Children Who Hate*. Glencoe, IL: Free Press.
Redl, F. & Wineman, D. (1952) *Controls From Within*. Glencoe, IL: Free press.
Redl, F. *When We Deal With Children*. (1966) Glencoe, IL: Free Press.
Wineman, D. (1959) The Life Space Interview, *Social Work 4* (1) Pgs. 3-17.

What Fritz Redl Taught Me About Aggression: Understanding the Dynamics of Aggression and Counteraggression in Students and Staff

Nicholas J. Long, PhD

The American University

EDITOR'S NOTE: The astounding increase in the prevalence and intensity of youthful aggressive behavior is the prime challenge to all who work with children and youth. No area of behavior is less adequately handled by adults. Long builds on what Redl taught him concerning the dynamics of aggression. Out of Long's extensive experience in training professionals to cope with aggression has come the Conflict Cycle Paradigm. This paper provides specific assistance for hygienic response to the onslaught of aggressive behavior.

In most religions, caring for the needy is described as a necessary, rewarding and uncomplicated experience. Caring for others involves the simple process of personal giving. For example, if a child is hungry, you feed him. If a child is cold, you clothe him. If a child is tired, you provide him with a place to rest, and if he is lonely, you offer him your friendship. Under these helping conditions, the needy child usually is appreciative of your help, thanks you for your kindness, and leaves you with an enhanced feeling of altruism and self-worth. What makes this process of helping appealing is that it does not involve any specialized skills except for having a large and compassionate heart.

In 1956, when I worked for Fritz Redl at National Institute of Mental Health (N.I.M.H.), he presented a different view of helping to his staff. Fritz emphasized that helping aggressive students is not just a matter of love, dedication, and charity, but a complicated intra-psychic and interpersonal process involving many dynamic concepts and skills. For many of us, helping aggressive students, who had low frustration tolerance, rapid flights into panic and attack, few guilt feelings, exaggerated demands, a lack of realism and a denial of problem-solving skills was an overwhelming personal experience. I believe Fritz, however, loved aggressive students. He had that unique capacity to accept them at their very worst. In fact, he seemed to be at his best when he was in a crisis interview (life space interview: LSI) with them. During these times, Fritz's insights, wit, logic, timing, strength and reality tenderness were flawless, and those of us who observed him were instant admirers of his skills. As a result, Fritz left an enduring mark on his staff that never faded over time.

Fritz fathered many therapeutic concepts for residential treatment programs. The two concepts which were most helpful to me as a beginning professional and which are still prerequisites to being an effective helper with aggressive students are: (1) Helping Begins with Understanding Ourself, and (2) Helping Begins By Understanding the Dynamics of Aggression.

HELPING BEGINS BY UNDERSTANDING OURSELF

I recall hearing Fritz give a brilliant lecture to about 500 educators. He said, "As teachers we have a room, a group, equipment, materials, a curriculum, instructional methods, and grades; but most of all, we have ourselves. What happens to us emotionally in the process of teaching emotionally disturbed kids is the critical factor in determining our effectiveness." Fritz continued by emphasizing that there are no great teachers, psychologists, social workers, or child care counselors. He smiled and said, "There are not enough angels to go around, so ordinary people, like us, with our unique histories choose to work with emotionally disturbed kids."

He pointed out that there are many troubled students in our classrooms with whom we have an excellent psychological fit and as a result we feel comfortable and competent to help them. There are other students with whom the psychological fit is okay, but we will need professional support to maintain a helping relationship. He also believed there are a few students in every classroom or residential center who have the ability to stir up strong feelings in us. The intensity of these stirred-up feelings represents our unfinished social history or developmental conflicts. This becomes our personal and private psychological luggage which we carry with us on our daily travels.

Unfortunately, a few students seem to have the emotional keys to our psychological luggage and they seem to delight in exposing our "personal affairs" to everyone in the setting. As a result, these students are emotionally upsetting and difficult for us to help so we are likely to react to their attacks by calling them, "too sick for this program," "Crazy," "Bizarre," or "Psychotic." While name-calling may soothe our feelings temporarily, the reality of our profession demands that we acknowledge how our social history predetermines us to respond to select behaviors in specific ways.

OUR CONDITIONED REACTIONS
TO SELECT STUDENT BEHAVIOR

Let's take an incident in which a student starts crying during an LSI. What is our characteristic way of reacting to cry behavior? The answer lies somewhere in our early socializing experiences and what crying meant to us emotionally. Given six staff, their spontaneous reactions to crying could range from sympathy, sadness, detachment, bewilderment, embarrassment, to disgust and anger.

When working with aggressive students, the range of personal feelings that get stirred up in us is even greater than those generated by tears. For example, if we were raised by demanding authoritarian parents, alcoholic parents, primitive parents, or parents with episodic impulsive breakthroughs, we may grow up fearing aggression. When we are involved in any interpersonal situations involving aggressive behavior such as yelling, cursing, and threatening behaviors, the aggressive behavior may reactivate our childhood feelings of vulnerability and all we can think about is how to escape from this painful situation. In this scenario, we are likely to avoid setting limits with an aggressive student and to allow him too much leeway before stopping his inappropriate behavior.

Given the same social history, we may have solved our fear of aggression by learning a different solution to our feelings of vulnerability. Instead of running from aggression, we may identify with our aggressive parents and become like them. Frequently, this means as children we developed a personality characterized by a short emotional fuse with highly explosive behavior. As adults, our fear is that we will loose controls over our aggressive impulses and in a moment of anger end up doing something destructive to others. To manage this fear, the solution is to avoid "hot emotional situations" that could get us "out of control." If we work with aggressive students, the psychological fit between our need to stay in control and the student's lack of control becomes a central problem. In this scenario, we are likely to over control an aggressive student's behavior and to set rigid limits which provide no margin or tolerance for acting out.

The need to understand the relationship between our history and our perception of a current conflict with select students is not easy, but it is essential to our role and function as a therapeutic helper. Let me give you an example. Just recently I was supervising a graduate student (Patricia) who was complaining about the pleasure Jerome (a 12-year old student in our senior group at Rose School) seemed to take in teasing and intimidating Inez, a 7-year old girl in the youngest group. The more Pat talked about what she observed, the more vindictive she became toward Jerome. She said, "Behavior like Jerome's should never happen in a therapeutic school. It's not fair to Inez and Jerome shouldn't get away with his verbal abuse. He needs to be taught a lesson!" While I agreed that Jerome's behavior needed to be stopped, I also asked if this situation had a personal meaning to her since she seemed so upset by it. Pat looked puzzled and said, "No" and a few seconds later said, "Oh my God! It reminds me of what my older brother used to do to me when my parents weren't home."

Fritz was correct. Helping others does begin by understanding ourself and our unique developmental history.

HELPING BEGINS BY UNDERSTANDING THE DYNAMICS OF AGGRESSION

The other side of self-awareness is to understand the "Dynamics of the Aggressive Conflict Cycle" and how aggressive students can create in us their feelings and if we are not trained how they can cause us to mirror their aggressive behavior, *independent of our social history and personality.*

While aggressive behavior is driven by many different reasons, the dynamics of aggression is predictable. The aggressive student has never learned to tolerate normal amounts of frustration, disappointment or anxiety. Instead of owning these feelings, he gives them away by attacking or depreciating everyone in sight. He knows how to engage us by using words and/or actions which "push our emotional buttons." While these aggressive behaviors reduce the aggressive student's level of anxiety, his behavior simultaneously creates normal counteraggressive feelings in us. If we are not trained to understand the dynamics of aggression, we not only will pick up the students aggressive feelings but also we will behave in similar counteraggressive ways, thus escalating the conflict. For example, when a student shouts, "I'm not going to do it!" "Don't you hear me?!" We are likely to raise our voice and say, "You will do it!" "Do You Hear Me!" By mirroring the student behavior, we create more psychological stress in the student. The student's feelings become more intense, and his behavior becomes more primitive. At this point, we become locked into a power struggle with the student and will continue to escalate the problem beyond reason. At this moment, most of us, who are caught in this power struggle frequently say with triumphant resentfulness, "I would rather die than give in to this S.O.B. student." What's surprising about this Aggressive Conflict Cycle is that even if the student loses the power struggle and is suspended, or physically restrained, the aggressive student's basic assumptions that adults are hostile and that he has a right to be angry or "to get even" are reinforced. Clearly there are no winners in a power struggle with aggressive students.

THE CONFLICT CYCLE PARADIGM
(or, How Not to Struggle in a Power Struggle with Aggressive Children and Youth)

To understand why and how competent staff find themselves in such painful and unproductive struggles with aggressive students, the Conflict Cycle Paradigm was developed. This paradigm (see Figure 1) describes how the interaction between a student and a staff follows a circular process in which the attitudes, feelings, and

FIGURE 1. The Pupil's Conflict Cycle

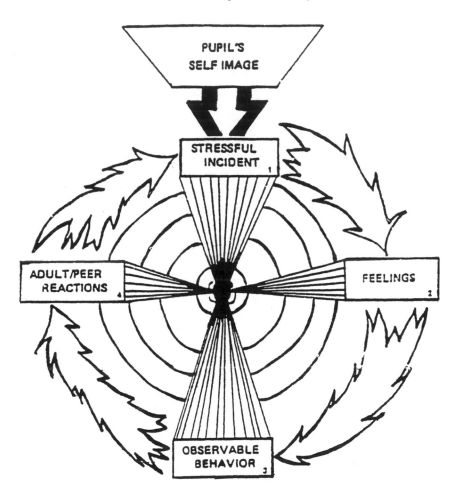

behaviors of the staff are influenced by and in turn influence the attitudes, feelings, and behaviors of the student. Once in operation, this negative interplay between student and staff is extremely difficult to interrupt. For example, we know that students under stress behave emotionally rather than rationally. They are controlled more by feelings than by logic. They protect themselves from physical and psychological pain by becoming defensive, primitive, and regressive. To understand the dynamics of the Aggressive Conflict Cycle, the following five circular steps are presented.

1. *Self-Concept:* A student's self-concept consists of his collected views and perceptions of himself and the kind of person he feels he is. This includes all of his values, beliefs, and images — whether he thinks he is bright or dull, mature or infantile, healthy or sick, friendly or fearful, attractive or unattractive, verbal or nonverbal, etc. What a student believes about himself is more important in determining his behavior than is any score on an objective test.

   A central part of the self-concept of any emotionally disturbed student is the development of his self-fulfilling prophecy. This is his characteristic way of perceiving, feeling, thinking, and behaving that helps him manage his psychological pain. Just as a primitive tribe tries to interpret the destructive power of cosmic forces such as tidal waves or volcanoes as due to something the tribe has done to offend the gods, troubled children have to explain to themselves a life of neglect, physical abuse, unrealistic expectations, and loss. The search for an explanation is necessary for their adjustment. Unfortunately, their attempts to make sense out of their bizarre and incongruent life result in naive and rigid cognitive conclusions. Frequently, they result in such internalized attitudes as:

   "I'm not worthy of love — so don't get close."

   "Never trust or be dependent on adults if you are going to get your needs met."

   "The world is too dangerous to manage alone, so I need to find someone to rescue me."

   "Anger is dangerous and destructive, so I must never let people know what I am feeling."

   The self-fulfilling prophecy of "never trust or need adults" is the basic assumption of the highly aggressive student's power struggle and becomes active every time a staff initially tries to relate to him in a positive, supportive, and consistent way.

2. *Stress:* Stress is a subjective reaction to external conditions that are real, anticipated, or imagined and that cause physiological and/or psychological discomfort. Four different types of precipitating events have been identified as causes of varying degrees of stress:

   • *Physical stress* — for example, lack of food, water, sleep, elimination, or activity.
   • *Psychological stress* — for example, situations that lead to personal threats, acts of rejection, severe conditions of competition, boredom, conflict between two positive or negative alternatives, and unrealistic aspirations and standards.
   • *Reality stress or unplanned events* — for example, losing or breaking objects, being unavoidably delayed, having an accident, experiencing a traumatic event or a personal disappointment.
   • *Developmental stress* — for example, meeting new people, going to new places, separating from friends and settings, taking physical and academic examinations, being responsible for one's behavior at an appropriate developmental level.

   Factors influencing the impact of stress on the self-concept are the *duration, frequency, intensity,* and *multiplicity* of stress. For example, stress related to lack of sleep is different from the stress experienced when one simultaneously lacks sleep, is criticized by the teacher, tears his coat on a nail, and fails a math exam.

3. *Feelings:* Unfortunately, many students are taught that certain feelings or emotions are unacceptable. When these students experience these unacceptable feelings, they can't tolerate them so they find ways of getting rid of them by using a host of defense mechanisms such as denial, projection, displacement, rationalization, regression, etc.

   Also, students need to distinguish between their feelings and their behavior. For example, it is healthy to feel anger when one has been psychologically depreciated or cruelly discriminated against, although it is not acceptable to assault the offender. It is healthy to experience fear when someone threatens to hurt or abuse you, but it is not helpful to encourage it to happen. It is healthy to experience intense feelings of sadness when someone you love dies or moves away, but it is not healthy to withdraw from all relationships. It is healthy to feel guilty when you behave in a way you know is unacceptable, but it is not useful to act out so that others will punish you. It is normal to experience anxiety when you are anticipating a new experience or a new relationship, but it is not healthy to handle this anxiety by drinking or by using drugs. The existence and importance of accepting these feelings are incontestable. As Fritz said, "There is a difference between having feelings and being had by your feelings. If your feelings flood you, then your behavior becomes out of control."

4. *Observable Behavior:* When students react to feelings of stress by expressing them directly or by defending against them, they usually create additional problems for themselves in their milieu. Behaviors such as hitting, running away, stealing, teasing, lying, becoming hyperactive, fighting, using drugs, inattention, and withdrawal cause students to have difficulty with *teachers*, *peers*, *learning*, and *rules*. For example, when a student displaces his feelings of hostility he has toward his mother on the staff, an inevitable staff-student problem develops. If this interpretation of behavior is accepted, staff can understand that many of the problems students cause in treatment programs are not always the causes of their problems. More accurately, the problems students cause in residential centers are frequently the result of the way they have learned to cope with their feelings of stress. For students to understand why they behave in certain ways, they need to know how their feelings drive their behavior.

5. *Staff Reaction:* One of the amazing concepts of interpersonal relationships is that students in stress can actually generate their feelings and, at times, their behavior in others. For example, an aggressive student can quickly bring out hostile feelings and counter-aggressive behaviors in others. A hyperactive student can make others feel anxious and act in impulsive, irrational ways. Similarly, a detached student frequently gets

others to feel depressed and to ignore him. If staff are unaware of this natural reaction, the student's inappropriate behavior will become reinforced and perpetuated automatically by the teacher's reaction. The phrase, "Do unto others as others do unto you" is an accurate but unfortunate psychological consequence of the Conflict Cycle.

For example, the negative feedback a student receives from the staff frequently supports the student's original view of himself and his world, increasing his feelings and causing the student to behave in a more unacceptable and primitive way. As the student's behavior deteriorates, the staff becomes even more angry and disgusted with him. Consequently, the staff reacts in a negative, punitive way which is perceived by the student as more rejection, intensifying his stress, feelings, and behavior. The conflict cycle continues around and around until an intense power struggle develops between the staff and the student. During these cycles, logic, caring, and compassion vanish, and the only goal is to win the power struggle. For staff, the student is seen as the source of the problem. He is told to "shape up" and to improve his attitude and behavior.

There are no winners when the Aggressive Conflict Cycle reaches the level of the power struggle. This cycle cannot be broken by asking students in stress to act maturely during intense states of conflict. If change is going to occur, *the staff must accept the primary responsibility for acting in a mature and in a professional manner.*

This assumes that staff are aware of how students in stress will try to provoke them to act in impulsive, dispassionate, and rejecting ways. Once staff knows in advance what these students are trying to do to them, this knowledge gives them a professional advantage. To be forewarned is to be forearmed. The staff's struggle is not to be baited or seduced into a power struggle, but to help aggressive students own their feelings and to be responsible for their behavior. Once this concept of not fighting with these students is accepted, specific intervention skills to prevent or break the Aggressive Conflict Cycle become useful.

BREAKING THE AGGRESSIVE CONFLICT CYCLE

To break the destructive force of Aggressive Conflict Cycle, the following concepts and techniques are offered to the Staff:

1. Conflict is to be viewed as a natural and inevitable part of the student's life.
2. Conflict is neither good or bad for a student but a function of the student's perceptions and thoughts.
3. During conflict, most students are flooded by their feelings (emotions).
4. During conflict, feelings usually drive a student's behavior which frequently is irrational, distorted and inappropriate causing problems with adults, peers, rules and learning.
5. During conflict, students are their worst enemy and will defend, deny, blame, rationalize and regress from owning their behavior or having responsibility for their behavior.
6. As a result, students in conflict frequently create in others their feelings, and if the staff is not trained, the staff may not only pick up the student's feeling but also may mirror the student's inappropriate behaviors.
7. If The Aggressive Conflict Cycle follows its normal pattern, the initial stressful incident becomes escalated into a new and painful "power struggle" in which there are no winners.

CHANGING THE AGGRESSIVE CONFLICT CYCLE TO A COPING CYCLE

The following concepts and skills are offered to the staff:

1. A knowledge of the Aggressive Conflict Cycle raises your consciousness about conflict since you know in advance that a student in stress will create in you his/her feelings. "To be forewarned is to be forearmed."
2. A knowledge of the Aggressive Conflict Cycle enables you to accept and "own" your "counter aggressive feelings" toward this student as being genuine as well as providing a useful indicator of how *the student* is "feeling."
3. A knowledge of the Aggressive Conflict Cycle enables you to

own your counter aggressive feelings. This does not mean you deny them or act them out. Accepting your feelings begins by acknowledging that feelings exist to enrich your life and not to restrict your life. Personal insight comes when you can say "yes" to acknowledging your feelings and "no" to the expression of your counter aggressive feelings in behaviors which infringe on the "right of others." Thus, both parts of your life can live in harmony and not in conflict with each other—i.e., the intra-psychic, emotional, covert part of your life and your behavioral, rational, overt part.

4. A knowledge of the Aggressive Conflict Cycle helps you to *choose* not to struggle in a Power Struggle with this student. (a conscious choice—"I will not fight with you.")

5. A knowledge of the Aggressive Conflict Cycle helps you *stop* all "You" messages, which escalate the Aggressive Conflict Cycle. (i.e., "You apologize." "You better use your head.")

6. A knowledge of the Aggressive Conflict Cycle helps you to use "I" messages as a way of expressing your feelings while reducing the pressure of your "Double Struggle"—i.e., controlling your own feelings (fear of loss of self-control) while simultaneously trying to manage this student's inappropriate behaviors and intense feelings.

7. A knowledge of the Aggressive Conflict Cycle helps you to focus your energies on what a student *needs* instead of on what you are *feeling*.

8. A knowledge of the Aggressive Conflict Cycle helps you to remember that while feelings are real and powerful, they may not reflect an accurate assessment of the interpersonal conflict. Specifically, feelings are not a cognitive function and should not be used to determine what is helpful to this student at this particular time.

9. A knowledge of the Aggressive Conflict Cycle enables you to decode a student's behavior into his feelings.

10. A knowledge of the Aggressive Conflict Cycle enables you to help the student make the connection between his behavior, his feelings and the original stressful incident.

11. A knowledge of the Aggressive Conflict Cycle enables you to

help the student focus on managing stress, coping skills, the here and now, personal responsibility and self-worth.

Fritz' contributions to helping aggressive children and youth will be timeless. He had the rare ability to translate complicated ideas into understandable knowledge and functional skills.

I feel honored to have worked with him briefly and to promote his concepts of "Helping Begins By Understanding Ourself" and "Helping Begins By Understanding the Dynamics of Aggression."

Back to the Future:
Effective Residential Group Care and Treatment for Children and Youth and the Fritz Redl Legacy

Jerome Beker, EdD

University of Minnesota

EDITOR'S NOTE: In the tradition of Redl's vigorous advocacy papers, Beker examines the current "holiness game" of damning inpatient treatment on the basis of ideology, cost, assumed abuse and effectiveness. He reviews Redl's position on the potential of such settings and proposes that we look at new possible ingredients for residential work coming from his extensive experience in therapeutic camping.

On a variety of interrelated grounds, and not without some justification, residential group care and treatment programs for children and youth have been under attack for several decades. As a result, many such programs have been closed, often without viable alternatives in place, and others have been severely curtailed. Yet the numbers of young people in residential group care settings have, after a brief pause around the mid-eighties, apparently resumed their seemingly inexorable upward climb (Children's Defense Fund, 1990; Select Committee, 1989). In light of (1) the continuing scenario of family disintegration, with increasing numbers of addicted and other children growing toward adolescence without families even minimally equipped to deal with the challenges of normal child rearing, and (2) the unavailability of stable, supportive family foster placements for most such children, it does not appear likely that the need for such services will decline in the foreseeable future.

57

GROUP CARE AS PARIAH

Currently, placement outside the home, particularly in group care, is widely viewed as representing a failure of the system involved (usually, child welfare), rather than as the targeted use of one of a continuum of legitimate intervention options that can enhance a young person's life situation and, perhaps, that of his or her family. Why, in the face of our accelerating need as a society for all the childrearing help we can get, particularly for those young people whose natural families seem unable to meet their needs, have residential group care and treatment programs fallen into such disrepute, and what can we do about it? There appear to be at least four factors involved—ideology, perceived costs, presumed abuse, and results in terms of program effectiveness—each of which is considered briefly below.

Ideology

Based on his extensive, cross-national research on group care, Wolins (1974) has specified what appear to be six "ingredients of success" in such programs. All reflect ideological predispositions with which, he points out, many Americans may tend to have difficulty. More recently, Wells (in press) has reviewed and reinforced this observation in the context of the need for group care and our resistances to it in the 1990s. Thus, residential programs start out on the defensive, and to advocate for them is to make oneself vulnerable to the charge that his or her values are somehow outdated and/or otherwise flawed.

Costs

Residential programs certainly "look" more expensive; whether they actually are depends on the specifics of each program, on what they are compared to and, most importantly, on long-term calculations. Thus, for example, a successful residential group care or treatment program is certainly more cost effective over time than a nonresidential program that fails, leaving its charges as lifelong burdens (rather than contributors) to our society. In appropriate cases, higher daily costs of group care can even be offset by shorter intervention periods. But it seems that many of our fellow citizens and our decision makers tend to reject such longer-term perspectives, even with regard to more concrete preventive public health proposals with established effectiveness, so this argument seems unlikely to make much headway.

Paradoxically, the mechanisms that have been developed to pay for residential services — primarily, purchase-of-service arrangements by various governmental agencies and private insurers — have contributed to increasing costs through their adherence to sometimes inappropriate, medically oriented standards and requirements and through other measures ostensibly linked to quality control, the avoidance of liability exposure, and the like. Such practices may even preclude implementing the least restrictive, most effective program approaches and, in terms of the point at issue here, often tend to add significantly to costs.

It remains for those responsible for residential programs to pursue a dual approach to insure that the needed resources will be available. On the cost side, it is important to economize wherever possible, making the case that effective programming may not always be the most expensive and that extraneous, often medically-based staffing and procedural requirements may not contribute much to program effectiveness. On the resource side, evidence of short- and long-term cost effectiveness must be imbedded in efforts to educate decision makers and the citizenry in general as to the importance of the entire continuum of care and of residential services as appropriately applied in that context.

The Assumption of Abuse

Not unrelated to the ideological considerations raised above is the frequent characterization of residential group care and treatment programs as inherently abusive. Even where there is no "active" physical or emotional abuse, it is maintained, those in residential placement are abused passively by being deprived of freedom, of a family setting, of needed emotional support, of long-term relationships with loving adults, and the like. One need not deny that many of our residential programs have failed to serve the best interests of the young people in their care to observe that these presumed deficits are not intrinsic; rather, they reflect limited vision in program development, inadequate implementation, and/or broader (e.g., familial) factors extrinsic to the residential setting.

Nor does this reflect an anti-family bias; virtually all responsible professionals would prefer to sustain the family intact when that is a viable option and would look with favor on promising family foster care possibilities. Realistically, however, there are many times when such arrangements are not available or do not offer what is needed, and residential group care is (or should be) designed to fill that gap. Real tradeoffs may be required, e.g., in some aspects of freedom, but it is the responsibility of professionals, in concert with the young person involved and his or her family to the extent that that is feasible, to make such decisions in the light of the total situation.

For those who are deemed to require residential group care placements, we have the obligation to provide as well as we can — at the very least, a better situation overall than they would be likely to have at home — or out-of-home placement cannot be justified (G. Thomas, 1982). (The same consideration, incidentally, is appropriate for any proposed intervention in relation to any less restrictive option.) As to the argument that strengthening residential group care options tends to subvert efforts to promote less drastic alternatives, one can reply that to sacrifice on this basis the welfare of young people for whom there are no better alternatives would be unacceptable. Rather, the task is to strengthen family-based and other approaches at the same time.

Program Effectiveness

It seems clear that, as a whole, existing residential group care programs do not provide a panacea for most troubled and at-risk young people who cannot be served effectively in family frameworks. Moreover, most studies agree that what happens within such settings has less of an influence on outcomes than do such factors as the nature and extent of the problem that led to placement, and the success of post-placement integration in a caring, appropriate living and work or study context (Whittaker, Overstreet, Grasso, Tripodi, & Boylan, 1988). Thus, there is very little hard data showing that such programs can make a positive difference as that is measured by recidivism rates and the like, and there are clear (albeit largely anecdotal) indications that they can be abusive and harmful. As a result, some (e.g., Perrow, 1963, 1966) favor the development of residential facilities as benevolent custodial settings rather than aspiring to develop them as arenas for intensive treatment.

As in other fields, the search for new technologies that can solve operational problems has been felt in recent decades in residential group care. Behavior modification using point and level systems, for example, has become widespread in such settings, as has "positive peer culture" using guided group interaction and related methods. More managerially oriented administrative approaches have been applied in an effort to enhance economy and accountability. Despite some positive outcomes in terms of staff consistency in applying the operative models and their apparent treatment effects, however, such innovations have not broadly enhanced the image of residential group care, nor do they appear to have had much impact on its overall effectiveness. And the calls for its abolition do not seem to diminish, despite the fact that, at least for many young people, there do not appear to be any viable alternatives.

TOWARD A MORE PRODUCTIVE RESIDENTIAL MODEL

The concept of the "therapeutic milieu" is a familiar one in the history of residential treatment, its prominence in this connection dating perhaps from its exposition by Bettelheim and Sylvester (1948) over 40 years ago. The work of Redl and Wineman (1957, reprinting their writings of the early 1950s) at Pioneer House certainly reflected that notion, but it was not until years later that Redl (1958, 1959a) published his thinking on it explicitly in detail, including the use of the "life-space interview" (Redl, 1959b). A decade later, Trieschman (1969) added his insights, and program models based on this perspective proliferated throughout that period.

It was Redl, however, who most clearly articulated the therapeutic milieu idea with a normalizing, developmental perspective in ways that can be directly applied as criteria for effective practice. Dissecting the concept into its "seven most common meanings,"

Redl (1966) included at least four that he explicitly grounded in the developmental needs of all, not just troubled, children and youth, as follows:

1. *"Don't Put Poison in Their Soup"*

This refers to not doing to children and youth in residential programs what one ". . . wouldn't do to people anyway—any people—and [figuratively] to keep injurious substances out of their diets" (p. 72).

2. *"You Still Have to Feed Them"*

An extension of the preceding item to accentuate the positive, this refers to "basic-need coverage":

> They also bring with them all the other "basic human needs" of a given person in a given developmental phase with a given cultural background, regardless of whether or not such basic needs are closely related to the problems for which they were sent or even have anything to do with them. (p. 73)

Thus, such programs have the obligation to their clients

> . . . to see that their psychological nourishment contains all the [figurative] vitamins individuals of a given age need—beside the [figurative] medication administered for specific subgoals. (p. 73)

Redl does not suggest

> . . . that 'basic-need-coverage' in itself will bring about the desired therapeutic change. It is, rather, that, without its guaranteed provision, the intended therapy will be counteracted or that damage in other areas of the patient's life will be produced while we are busy blindly treating the one for which he was admitted. (p. 74)

It should also be noted that, in cases where placement has been made for situational reasons not involving dysfunctional responses on the part of the young person, little additional or specialized "therapeutic" intervention may be required, and to overprescribe in this area — as in others — can be counterproductive.

3. *"Developmental-Phase Appropriateness and Cultural-Background Awareness"*

> The very style of adult-child relationships that is normally expected to convey the impression of "cared-forness" and warmth is quite different for a five-year-old than, for instance, for an adolescent. . . . subcultural and other differences . . . complicate the issue even further. (pp. 74-75)

4. *"Re-Education for Life"*

Here, Redl speaks to the need to develop and maintain the vital connection between the young person in group care and the outside world — the family and the community — and his or her ability to live comfortably in it:

> . . . we are not satisfied with the appropriateness of the milieu for the present repair job to be done. We also want it to contain enough of the ingredients that the later, normal, open life situation will contain and to which the patient will have to adjust after his release. . . . We consider a milieu "therapeutic" only if it aspires to "outlive itself" and if it builds in . . . as many life experiences as the patient will have to meet later, hopeful that their taste may whet his appetite for more normal living rather than be obliterated by the smell of psychological determinants so importantly surrounding him now. (p. 79)

Recognizing the implicit paradox here — the need for providing both a specialized and a normalizing environment — Redl responds by proposing a progression of appropriate experiences that may take place in a range of settings, essentially the very current concept of the continuum of care. These perspectives, whether applied directly in the development of new program options or more subtly in enhancing existing programs, may point the way to more successful group care in the context of current needs and attainable resources.

PROGRAMMATIC APPROACHES TO NORMALIZATION

Thus, Redl (1966) presents us with the notion of normalization and the case for it in a nutshell. He goes further in other of his writings, looking to the developmental potency of environments that have been created for children and youth without special difficulties, such as schools and, most pertinent to the present discussion, residential summer camps. His thinking with regard to applying normalizing models in working with troubled and troubling children was not dissimilar to that of Hobbs (1966), which led to the development of the Re-ED programs that have had a broad impact on thinking in this field.

Awareness of the apparent potential of camping as a modality for working effectively with troubled children and youth had earlier led to the establishment of camps explicitly designed for a therapeutic mission, perhaps beginning with the University of Michigan Fresh Air Camp in 1921 (Lyman, 1981). Later, Redl joined with others, notably including Bill Morse, in building that program from its rudimentary beginnings into a sophisticated milieu treatment modality as well as a research and training laboratory that produced a steady flow of new knowledge (e.g., McNeil, 1957) and a generation of scholars and practitioners who have gone on to contribute to the broader field in a variety of significant ways. Camp Wediko, started in the late 1930s under the sponsorship of the Judge Baker Guidance Clinic in Boston, and the Dallas Salesmanship Club Camp (Loughmiller, 1965), started in the late 1940s, are two other widely recognized examples (Lyman, 1981). Among the largest current programs of this kind is that sponsored by the Eckerd Foundation at five locations in Florida.

Almost half a century ago, Redl (1942) chaired an American Camping Association workshop (supported by the W. K. Kellogg Foundation) on "The Role of Camping in Education." A few years later, he made more explicit his views about "the tremendous value of camping, educationally and also as a means of therapy" and articulated some of the opportunities as well as the risks of that medium, both of which are particularly pertinent to what we now call vulnerable children (Redl, 1947; see also pertinent articles listed and those reprinted in Redl, 1966). The maxim, "First, do no harm," implicit in his writings in this area, would seem to be an appropriate cautionary note in all our efforts with these young people (e.g., Redl, 1947). Bill Morse (Personal communication, June 1990) reports that disturbed boys could not be constructively maintained in such settings unless they brought at least two of the following three characteristics with them: a capacity for enjoyment; gratification in being with their peers; and the ability to "use" adult assistance. Having a significant vocational component also appeared to be crucial (see also Morse, 1957). Such observations have obvious implications for work with youth in other group care settings as well.

In recent decades, however, we seemed to forget much of what we had learned during the preceding period, in the face of increasing technological sophistication, incidence and severity of problem behavior, legal and fiscal accountability requirements, and other societal changes as we moved toward greater formalization of programs for and techniques used with troubled children and youth. Interestingly, much of Europe responded to similar challenges differently, in part by going back to some of the earlier American experiences discussed here, in the development of the *educateur* (variously named in different countries) as a generalist milieu practitioner (Barnes & Bourdon, 1990; Beker & Barnes, 1990).

In the United States, there has been an even more recent return to some of the kinds of ideas discussed above, in the development and application of which Redl played such a fundamental role, although now in a somewhat different context (Arieli, Beker, & Kashti, 1990). Three interrelated concepts have emerged as core ideas in this connection, each of which can be seen as integral to the camp milieu as Redl and others saw it, and each of which has significant implications for enhancing contemporary group care programs in general: challenge, participation, and service.

Challenge

Young people need to try their wings in various ways in the real world; boring programs without active challenge not only tend to dull and deaden their sensitivities (as they do ours), but also lead many of them to find their own excitement, often in ways that have gotten them into trouble in the past. Camping pioneer L. G. Sharp has observed in this connection that if we do not fill children's days with opportunities to do things that are fun, exciting, and good for them, they will fill their days with activities that are fun, exciting, and *not* good for them (or, it might be added, for us). A fundamental programming responsibility of those who work with youth in such settings is to make appropriate, constructive, and challenging options available and known to them.

At least for many young people, one essential element in challenge appears to be risk-taking, as is reflected in the kinds of wilderness and other adventure-based rehabilitative programs that have been expanding rapidly in recent years (Bacon & Kimball, 1989). Much progress has been made in the containment of physical risk in such experiences, without unduly diluting their excitement-potential, through activity design and standards for the training and performance of adult leaders. Likewise, ways to manage liability problems that such activities sometimes entail have begun to emerge. The Association for Experiential Education is among the groups that have been in the forefront of efforts in this direction, and at least one state has, with federal assistance, developed detailed standards for adventure programs in residential care (New Jersey, 1989).

Participation

The camp milieu is conceived as a community in which everyone involved has an ownership stake and a role. This is in contrast to the larger society, where young people frequently feel unwanted, unneeded, and socially impotent. It is in even starker contrast to many group care settings, where their role is even more passive: they are there essentially to have something done *to* them, to be "treated," rather than to reach out, to expand their horizons, and to grow. When a setting emphasizes the latter group of expectations, youth can be empowered developmentally, but this depends on their having a share in the important decisions and the core experiences that make a community what it is, thus making it theirs (Beker, 1989; Levy, in press; B. Thomas, in press; Wells, in press; Wolins,

1974). Camp—and other residential group settings—provide the potential for building just such an environment.

Service

The concept of service relates closely to participation, taking it a step farther. Making the community theirs implies that they share responsibility for it, for the welfare of all its members, and for doing the tasks that need to be done to sustain and build it. Such involvement also tends to build self-esteem. The camp milieu lends itself to and, in some respects, even requires such activities, both within and in relation to the larger, surrounding community, which often include work that is needed to maintain and improve the quality of life.

In many other contemporary residential settings, however, such work expectations for residents are viewed as exploitive, or at least as something to be avoided due to union sensitivities, legal exposure, and the like (Beker & Durkin, 1989). These are real issues that cannot prudently be minimized, and cases of exploitation are not unknown, but neither can we responsibly ignore the importance of providing such service learning opportunities for young people in out-of-home care, where they are particularly important in building feelings of connectedness, as Redl and others have emphasized. Such programs have been described by, among others, Barnes (in press) and Brendtro (1985).

IMPLICATIONS FOR RESIDENTIAL GROUP CARE PROGRAMS

The implications of the above may be drawn on three levels. Most concretely, the development of more camp-type placement options within the spectrum of group care services, where possible, seems to be worthy of consideration. More broadly, existing conventional residential group care programs, many of which already offer short-term camp experiences to their residents, might wish to add or expand such opportunities and to orient them, insofar as is practicable, in the directions suggested above. Finally, group care settings of all kinds can examine their regular, ongoing programs to determine how it might be possible to build in some of the community and other elements, described above, that emerge on the basis of the thinking of Redl and the others as essential.

These are not simple matters. McNeil (1957) and Redl (1947) are among those who have pointed out the developmental risks of such approaches. All require sensitive, knowledgeable staff leadership, particularly given the nature of most group care populations, which requires that (at least at the beginning) much of the impetus for fun and participation, much of the energy, must come from the staff. Yet many programs have been able to do it, and the precedents and approaches are available (see, e.g., Arieli, Beker, & Kashti, 1990; Bacon & Kimball, 1989; Barnes, in press; Durkin, 1988; Durkin, Forster, & Linton, 1989; Levy, in press; Loughmiller, 1965; Morse, 1957). The enthusiasm born of conviction that it can succeed is also an essential element (Beker & Feuerstein, 1989; Wolins, 1974).

CONCLUSION

There should be no dispute about the desirability of maintaining families intact whenever that is possible without hurting those involved. The development of family-and home-based services in recent years (Bryce, 1988) is a welcome innovation in that direction, although limitations (at least as such programs are currently being implemented) are also becoming evident (Summary, 1989; Wald, 1988). However, the magnitude of needs that do not appear to be amenable to in-home services is overwhelming. These include, for example, those represented by abandoned children (e.g., the increasing numbers of AIDS orphans), by children whose problems are so great as to be unmanageable even by marginally adequate parents with help (e.g., some addicted children), and by parents so debilitated by drugs or other factors as to be virtually nonfunctional in that role or intractably abusive (Ladner, 1990; Wells, in press).

The extent of these problems—current and anticipated—has led to calls for a new look at out-of-home care as a legitimate option (e.g., Wald, 1988) and even for expanded group residential services including orphanages (e.g., Ladner, 1990; Levy, in press; Wells, in press). If such services are predefined as representing failure, there will be little we can do to rescue the young people involved or to preserve our own professional self-respect. It should also be acknowledged that our track record in providing creative, effective, developmentally empowering work in the milieu has not been as convincing as we might wish.

In this connection, it has been noted above that group care challenges some typical American ideological notions, but success is also an American value; to the extent that we can demonstrate effective work, the pragmatism that seems to be part of our national character can prevail to rekindle public interest and support. By revisiting the perspectives that were elaborated by Redl and his colleagues in an earlier decade, and in the context of more recent thinking about their programmatic implications (including the possibility of increased family involvement, e.g., Aldgate, 1987; Carman & Small, 1988), we can recapture our own excitement and, thus, reinvigorate our capacity to serve the developmental needs of troubled children and youth effectively.

REFERENCES

Aldgate, J. (1987). Residential care: A reevaluation of a threatened resource. *Child and Youth Care Quarterly*, *16*, 48-59.

Arieli, M., Beker, J., & Kashti, Y. (1990). Residential group care as a socializing environment: Toward a broader perspective (pp. 45-58). In J. Anglin, C. Denholm, R. Ferguson, & A. Pence (Eds.), *Perspectives in professional child and youth care*. New York: The Haworth Press, Inc. (Also published as a special issue of *Child & Youth Services*, *13*(1).)

Bacon, S. B., & Kimball, R. (1989). The wilderness challenge model. In R. D. Lyman, S. Prentice-Dunn, & S. Gabel (Eds.), *Residential inpatient treatment of children and adolescents*. New York: Plenum.

Barnes, F. H. (in press). From warehouse to greenhouse: Play, work, and the routines of daily living in groups as the core of milieu treatment. In J. Beker & Z. Eisikovits (Eds.), *Knowledge utilization in residential child and youth care practice*. Washington, DC: The Child Welfare League of America.

Barnes, F. H., & Bourdon, L. (1990). Cross-cultural perspectives in residential youthwork: The French educateur and the American child care worker (pp. 301-315). In J. P. Anglin, C. Denholm, R.V. Ferguson, & A. Pence (Eds.), Perspectives in professional child and youth care work. New York: The Haworth Press, Inc. (Also published as a special issue of *Child & Youth Services*, *13*(2).)

Beker, J. (1989). On building community. *Child and Youth Care Quarterly*, *18*(2), 79-80.

Beker, J., & Barnes, F. H. (1990). The educateur returns to America: Approaching the development of professional child and youth care cross-culturally through ILEX. *Child and Youth Care Quarterly, 19*(3).

Beker, J., & Durkin, R. P. (1990). The role of work in residential group care programs for children and youth. St. Paul, MN: Center for Youth Development & Research, Univ. of Minnesota.

Beker, J., & Feuerstein, R. (1989). Toward a common denominator in effective group care programming: The concept of the modifying environment. Jerusalem: Hadassah-WIZO-Canada Research Institute.

Bettelheim, B., & Sylvester, E. (1948). A therapeutic milieu. *American Journal of Orthopsychiatry, 18,* 191-206.

Brendtro, L. K. (1985). Making caring fashionable: Philosophy and procedures of service learning. *Child Care Quarterly, 14,* 4-13.

Bryce, M. E. (1988). Family-based services; Preventive intervention (pp. 177-203). In D. H. Olson (Ed.), *Family-based perspectives in child and youth services.* New York: The Haworth Press, Inc. (Also published as a special issue of *Child & Youth Services, 11*(1).)

Carman, G. O., & Small, R. W. (Eds.). (1988). *Permanence and family support: Changing practice in group child care.* Washington, DC: Child Welfare League of America.

Children's Defense Fund. (1990). *A Children's Investment Agenda for 1990.* Washington, DC: Author.

Durkin, R. (1988). A competency-oriented summer camp and year round program for troubled teenagers and their families. *Residential Treatment for Children and Youth, 6*(1), 63-85.

Durkin, R., Forster, M., & Linton, T. E. (1989). The Sage Hill program for competency promotion. In E. A. Balcerzak (Ed.), *Group care of children: Transitions toward the year 2000.* Washington, DC: The Child Welfare League of America.

Hobbs, N. (1966). Helping disturbed children: Psychological and ecological strategies. *American Psychologist, 21,* 1105-1115. (Also in Wolins, 1974).

Ladner, J. (1990). Bring back the orphanages. *Family Therapy Networker, 14*(1), 48-49.

Levy, Z. (in press). Eagerly awaiting a home: A response from abroad. *Child and Youth Care Quarterly.*

Loughmiller, C. (1965). *Wilderness road.* Austin: Hogg Foundation for Mental Health, University of Texas.

Lyman, R. D. (1981). Non-institutional residential facilities for children and adolescents. In M. Dinoff & D. L. Jacobsen (Eds.), *Neglected problems in community mental health.* (pp. 58-65). Tuscaloosa, AL: Univ. of Alabama Press.

McNeil, E. B. (Ed.). (1957). Therapeutic camping for disturbed youth [Special Issue]. *The Journal of Social Issues, 13*(1).

Morse, W. C. (1957). An interdisciplinary therapeutic camp. *The Journal of Social Issues, 13*(1), 15-22.

New Jersey Department of Human Services, Division of Youth and Family Services. (1989). *Regulatory Module for Children's Residential Facilities that Provide Adventure Activities.* Trenton: Author.

Perrow, C. (1963). Reality shock: A new organization confronts the custody/ treatment dilemma. *Social Problems, 10,* 374-382.

Perrow, C. (1966). Reality Adjustment: A young institution settles for humane care. *Social Problems, 10,* 69-79.

Redl, F. (1942). Report of the workshop on the role of camping in education. *Camping Magazine, 14*(2), 41-43, 68-70.

Redl, F. (1947). Psychopathologic risks of camp life. *The Nervous Child, 6*(2), 139-147.

Redl, F. (1958). The meaning of "therapeutic milieu." *Symposium on Preventive and Social Psychiatry* (Walter Reed Army Institute of Research). Washington, DC: U. S. Government Printing Office.

Redl, F. (1959a). The concept of a "therapeutic milieu." *American Journal of Orthopsychiatry, 29,* 721-736. (Modified version in Redl, 1966.)

Redl, F. (1959b). Strategy and techniques of the life space interview. *American Journal of Orthopsychiatry, 29,* 1-18. (Modified version in Redl, 1966.)

Redl, F. (1966). *When we deal with children: Selected writings.* New York: Free Press.

Redl, F., & Wineman, D. (1957). *The aggressive child.* New York: Free Press. (Also published as *Children who hate,* 1951, and *Controls from within,* 1952. New York: Free Press.)

Select Committee on Children, Youth, and Families, U. S. House of Representatives. (1989). *No place to call home: Discarded children in America.* Washington, DC: U. S. Government Printing Office. November.

Summary of the Meeting on National Family Preservation. (1989). Charlotte, North Carolina, November 11-15. Unpublished manuscript.

Thomas, B. (in press). A response to "eagerly awaiting. . . . " *Child and Youth Care Quarterly.*

Thomas, G. (1982). The responsibility of residential placements for children's rights to development (pp. 23-45). In R. Hanson (Ed.), *Institutional abuse of children and youth.* New York: The Haworth Press, Inc. (Also published as a special issue of *Child & Youth Services, 4*(1/2).)

Trieschman, A. E. (1969). Understanding the nature of a therapeutic milieu. In A. E. Trieschman, J. K. Whittaker, & L. K. Brendtro (Eds.). *The other 23 hours: Child care work in a therapeutic milieu.* New York: Aldine.

Wald, M. S. (1988). Family preservation: Are we moving too fast? *Public Welfare, 46*(3). 33-38,46.

Wells, K. (in press). Eagerly awaiting a home: Severely emotionally disturbed youth, lost in our system of care—a personal reflection. *Child and Youth Care Quarterly.*

Whittaker, J. K., Overstreet, E. J., Grasso, A., Tripodi, T., & Boylan, F. (1988). Multiple indicators of success in residential youth care and treatment. *American Journal of Orthopsychiatry, 58,* 143-147.

Fritz Redl and Residential Treatment at Hawthorn Center

Ralph D. Rabinovitch, MD

Hawthorn Center, Northville, Michigan

EDITOR'S NOTE: In this charming tribute to Redl, Rabinovitch presents Redl as consultant, in this specific case to a state psychiatric hospital for children and adolescents. Some of Redl's most potent thoughts on milieu treatment are reviewed as well as the impact of these ideas on the program. But beyond that, Rabinovitch has captured for us the wit, humor and apt language which enabled Redl's expertise to be absorbed by his conferees.

In 1959, when he returned to Detroit from his work at the National Institute of Mental Health, we asked Fritz Redl to be our consultant on milieu treatment at Hawthorn Center. For 14 years, until he and Helen moved to Massachusetts, Tuesday was a red-letter day at Hawthorn. Fritz conducted seminars for multidiscipline staff and met with small groups or individuals to discuss special problems as they arose; as you would guess, they arose often.

Hawthorn Center is a large psychiatric hospital for children and adolescents located in Northville, Michigan. It is a State Department of Mental Health facility with inpatient, day treatment, outpatient, professional training and research units. When Fritz Redl was with us there were 150 inpatient beds and 100 additional children in the day treatment section. The age range was, and still is, 5 to 16 years. The living areas provide a broad range of facilities with much activity centered around the school. Fritz liked to spend time in the classrooms, the shops, the art rooms, the greenhouse, the work-study program, as well as the living units and he brought to the seminars many observations from these visits.

Fritz' first visit to Hawthorn Center was memorable. On the first

Tuesday when he came to my office, my secretary mistook him for the piano tuner whom we were also expecting that morning. She asked him if he wouldn't mind starting with the piano in cottage 2. As always Fritz rose to the occasion: "You won't believe it, but I forgot my instruments." I rescued Helen Richard and from then on she and Fritz were great friends. Fritz remembered the incident for years and often referred to it with that special sparkle that we so much enjoyed.

In this appreciation I plan to review some of Fritz Redl's thoughts on milieu treatment and their impact on the program at Hawthorn Center. But as I think back, another aspect of his life's work keeps intruding and I'd like to talk about this briefly first — his prodigious advocacy for children and programs for children. He never refused requests to enter a battle for a good cause. Who could ever forget those Redl speeches with their arresting and rousing language. "How to Mangle a Soul" and "Where Children Rot" date back to 1945. Later, for many years as a member of the Advisory Board of the Michigan Association for Emotionally Disturbed Children, he gave countless talks, all carefully prepared, on a whole range of "Crisis in the Children's Field" issues. He used to say that he did not know "a cure" for all the ills but that he tried to administer "emergency injections to a catatonic community to bring about at least temporary relief." How potent — and helpful — those injections were!

From its very beginning, and through all its 35 years to date, Hawthorn Center has had the good fortune to have had the direct involvement of many superb experts. Before the first child was admitted, Lauretta Bender helped define the clinical diagnostic emphases. From the first months, William Morse guided the establishment of the school for our children and our special education teacher-training program, and he is still actively involved. A little later, Fritz Redl led us to define our milieu treatment, and over the 14 years of his participation he helped us constantly to redefine it. More recently, Peter Blos, Jr., has been leading an ongoing seminar on individual psychotherapy.

In the Redl seminars, a vast range of topics relating to milieu were discussed; I can include here only a small, representative sampling. Fritz was a great linguist. I recall his charming, amused response when a student once asked him if he was planning to conduct his seminar that day in English, German, French or Redlese. He had a remarkable knack with words and the awesome flow of Redlese made the most difficult concepts graphic. The imagery and humor were truly unique. Often we had to work hard to follow his creative genius and sometimes we couldn't quite make it. But you can be sure there was never a dull or wasted moment. I have introduced each topic that follows with a phrase that Redl used in his discussions. I hope that they will give some flavor of his thinking, his style, and his teaching with its stress on crucial real-life issues.

SOME GENERAL PRINCIPLES

In Redl's criteria for a therapeutic milieu a number of general principles were crucial:

"Don't Put Poison in Their Soup"

An absolute sine qua non was a high standard of decent, benign, non-punitive care. In its absence there was no room for further discussion and rationalizing, through rhetoric, theorizing and philosophizing did not impress Redl. It was this practical, honest emphasis that energized his great social influence. On this crucial issue, as on many others, Redl never compromised.

"You Still Have to Feed Them"

Redl was always involved in the complex issue of integrating individual therapy into the total residential program. He of course recognized the contributions of individual psychotherapy but his heart was closer to the milieu. Regardless of the specific therapy needs of each child and the written plans to meet these needs, all the children are living in the unit 24-hours a day "and you'd better not forget it."

"It's More Like a Harem Than a Family"

At a time when the concept of the residential program as direct substitute family was popular, Redl stressed the need for diffusion and dilution of attachments between children and staff. At Hawthorn Center we have followed this design.[1] Each child has an individual therapist with whom he has a special relationship and who is his advocate, mediator and interpreter in the total program. But in the milieu there are no assigned substitute parents; attachments to staff occur spontaneously from a broad selection available to the child and these relationships are carefully monitored.

THE MILIEU STAFF

As expected, staff roles, responsibilities, rewards and related issues were recurring foci for discussion:

"After All, We're Only People"

Redl took it for granted, like everyone else, that "the most important aspect of a milieu is staff" and that many virtues in workers are desirable, including integrity, maturity, self-discipline and flexibility. He called the primacy of staff self-evident and, having mentioned the obvious, he rarely referred to it again. He hated cliches and avoided them. He did, however, give much attention to the questions of staff recruitment, selection and training. He always hoped for the ideal and expected the best. At the same time he recognized inevitable limitations; a major source of his profound influence with front-line workers was his respect for them as they were, with the prospect of continuing growth always implied.

"Let's All Bail Together, or Else"

The theme was the need for every worker to identify, beyond his or her individual discipline or points of view, with the total program. Either we keep the boat afloat together or we all sink together. This issue was especially crucial in a setting like ours with a very large staff drawn from at least eight disciplines. It was not always easy to maintain identification with the total effort but Redl kept the issue in the air and deftly brought us back to it.

"Prima Donna — So Long"

A specific related situation that especially intrigued Redl was the relationship of the individual therapists (psychiatrists, psychologists, and social workers in our setting) to the milieu program. He spotted with an eagle (and jaundiced) eye the therapists who viewed the milieu as an interfering ancillary, and they picked up the message loud and clear. Unreasonable territorial issues, rivalries, conflicting goals were often handled in the seminars with humor, directed not at the person but at the situation — a rare skill that was part of Redl's teaching genius.

"The Staff, Their Attitudes and Feelings — but Please Let's Not Call It All 'Transference'"

In the field in general it was customary to spend hours in at times racking discussions of workers' feelings; these topics were often raised in Redl's seminars. He acknowledged their importance and listened patiently for a while but before long managed to channel the discussion to issues of child management. Feelings are always present but a major challenge for the worker is to separate feelings from action, "two very different items on the milieu menu."

"Behavior Received in a Day's Time"

The impact of action or specific management is the focus here. There is a constant need to define the "forms" employed by staff for intervention — "limit-setting, expression of acceptance and love, etc.," — the actual communications to the child. Sensitivity to these forms is crucial for staff role awareness and monitoring. There is often a conflict between feeling and form. An interesting example arose from time to time in the overuse of snacks in the living areas. During these binges, wishing to provide compensatory gratification, everyone seemed to ply nourishment day and night. There was no question that many of the children at Hawthorn, previously deprived, needed compensatory gratification at many levels. But when gratification becomes seduction, a pause to examine the form of intervention is in order. Here the feeling, the wish to gratify, is positive; the form is negative. As Redl reminded us, pacifiers are usually at best only transiently effective.

"It's So Sensible, It's Amazing It Happened"

In 1956, with the inception of Hawthorn Center, we established the Civil Service category of child care worker, within the department of nursing. The child care workers were drawn, for the most part, from students (minimal requirement—two years of college completed with continuing enrollment) or recent graduates (bachelor's degree), usually in education, psychology, or social work. Through the years, from this staffing pattern, a professional cadre of senior child care supervisors has emerged and they have come to share milieu management responsibility with a group of psychiatric nurses, equally interested in milieu. Another group of nurses are "medical," and the overall department directors are our most senior psychiatric nurses. Redl appreciated and fostered the development of these milieu treatment professionals, drawn from a number of disciplines; he told us that it gave further proof that "evolution really works."

PROGRAMMING

Details of programming were always a major focus of Redl's concern; he was one of those rather rare consultants who move beyond generalities into the heart of a program. Year after year he explored a vast range of issues, one question suggesting another. A look at just a few of these should give some sense of the total:

"Strong Binding But Made of Elastic"

The need for structure, with rules and regulations, was assumed in the Redl philosophy and he had little sympathy for "a chaos stance," but it was structure with "elasticity"; the two words always went together. And the stress, when there was one, was usually on the side of the elasticity. At Hawthorn, with over 250 children (inpatient and day treatment) in our care, limits of tolerance had to be defined for a wide range of behaviors. Despite the fact that most of the children observed most of the limits most of the time, the day's program, carefully planned and scheduled, rarely reached evening in its original form. Blowups are unscheduled. A high degree of total staff energy goes into containment needs — self-defense, peace-keeping, arbitrating disputes. The efficiency, and in some cases the efficacy, of a program can be gauged by what we have come to call the T/S energy ratio where T is energy directed to treatment and S is energy directed to survival. When survival energy exceeds treatment energy, therapy goals are subverted and risk of staff exhaustion is high. Consideration of ways to lower the S factor was a frequent and vital seminar topic.

Among the rules there were always some absolute no-noes, such as no physical attacks on others, no destruction of furniture, no strongly offensive language. Redl approved the list with the comment "Good luck." And he liked to express feigned shock at the occasional bruise sustained by staff, the periodic broken chair, and the rich vocabulary that staff acquired.

"Different Ages, Different Needs, Different Problems"

In a program such as Hawthorn's, with as broad a range of age (5-16 years) and patient psychopathology, the issue of grouping in the living units is crucial. Our children are not grouped according to age or diagnosis; the spreads in each unit are wide. There are many advantages to this system. For the staff, the types of attention called for are diffused. For the children, ready-made models are available: the less-well-integrated tend to follow the more intact; the aggression-inhibited tend to identify with the more aggressive; the acting-out may try to emulate peers who stay out of trouble.

In this setting Redl had a special interest in the many and varied social groupings and activities that evolved spontaneously and their potential for use in the interest of particular children. Rather than try to create new opportunities artificially, workers were helped to recognize the times and ways to direct children into appropriate ongoing activities; these often provided more meaningful and rewarding involvements.

This is just one example of a myriad of aspects and nuances of the social structure of the milieu that Redl discussed, from pecking order to scapegoating to subclique formation to mascot-cultivation to — to — : creativity unending.

"The Reality of Time and Place; the Outspoken Behavior Expectation"

The concept of a general or overall behavior expectation is as illusory as it is undesirable. Different parts of the program have different ascribed expectations; children learn this early and find comfort in the assurances conveyed. At school a high level of attention and conformity is demanded. At mealtimes there is spontaneous conversation and fun but within an expectation of a reasonable decorum with prescribed rules. At free times in the living areas there is considerably more permissiveness. In some of the recreation activities on the premises the restrictions involve little beyond physical safety. On field trips a whole new set of social amenities is imposed. Redl considered as a strong research challenge balance in the distribution of these many program areas, selectively for different groups according to "developmental phase appropriateness."

"The Life Space Interview"

Sometimes after a disturbing experience, children need "first-aid services for the muddled feelings at the time." This intervention permits "a positive milieu impact"; without it, the impact may be quite negative. Redl gives as an example a child who is "running away unhappy, after a cruel razzing received from a thoughtless group." A friendly worker follows the child and, in the on-the-spot interview, comforts him. The result is a positive milieu impact.

At other times the life space interview may be used, shortly after the incident, to umpire quarrels or misunderstandings between two or more children. This application has led some workers to misinterpret the technique as an inquisitional third-degree procedure. Redl stressed the opposite — benign, insightful intervention by a sympathetic adult.

"The Value System That Oozes Out of Our Pores"

Children are remarkably aware of, and sensitive to the atmosphere of the treatment milieu — the attitudes that we have toward them and the expectations that we convey. At Hawthorn we have striven for a general tone that recognizes and accepts pathology, but also sets realistic goals and demands for gradual change. After a child has had an opportunity to experiment by testing the milieu, and after he has experienced warmth in relationships and established some trust, to permit negative patterns to continue unnecessarily in important areas is to miss the point of milieu treatment. When the child's readiness to move is recognized in the group living situation or the school, staff members work together to support and reinforce the growth.

To gauge how much to expect and when are critical challenges in milieu treatment. Realistic behavior expectations are an absolute necessity, but not always easy to define. Identified with our children and always hoping for the best for them, we may tend to set the goals too high. At other times we are afraid to demand enough. Pacing and the recognition of periods of growth and of plateaus are important. Each child's capacity for change and rate of movement are unique, and the clinical diagnosis provides only a general guideline for expectations. Detailed knowledge of the child's history and clinical realities, and sensitivity to his or her styles of interaction, are crucial.

Redl noted a wide range in individual worker's capacity to identify with these clinical subtleties; he called the factor "the clinical convictions of what is professionally correct handling." He recognized it gratefully in staff at every level of training, including some "questionnaire-clumsy workers on a low salary level."

This brief remembrance has, I hope, evoked some sense of the genius, the wit and the language of Fritz Redl and the magnitude of his clinical, social and teaching contributions. What a great heritage he has left us. And there is still another remarkable aspect of his thinking that finds repeated expression in his writings and speeches: "I would love to know." "This problem is far from solved." "I would like to find out more." "There is a great research challenge here." "Much more work needs to be done." "I am convinced of only one thing for sure — we all have quite a way to go."

Despite his prodigious expertise, this desire to learn more, to find new answers, to extend the boundaries of insight into disturbed children's treatment needs, is another great Fritz Redl legacy for all of us — and especially for today's young workers and those to come. In his writings they will find many seeds for the new knowledge-through-study that he so prized.

NOTE

1. References to the Hawthorn Center milieu program are drawn from The Program Outline, written and refined over the years by, among others, Drs. Sara Dubo, Harold L. Wright, Harold J. Lockett, Francis C. Pasley, Morris Weiss and James E. Galligan.

Consultation:
Redl's Influence

Ruth G. Newman, PhD

Private Practice: Washington, DC

EDITOR'S NOTE: While Ruth Newman was working with Redl on the NIMH project in Washington they together devised a 'learning experiment' on consultation. This article is derived from Newman's book on their specially funded project. As the paper illustrates, consultation Newman-Redl style is set in a new mold. While the setting in this instance was the school, the concepts apply to any milieu setting and is as important to those who engage consultants as those who consult.

While Redl was widely recognized for his consultation to child serving systems, the fact that he also turned his creative genius to developing a more vigorous style of consultation is not well known. To the best of my knowledge, he wrote no formal papers on the subject but he was involved in the study of consultation as a way to improve the milieu for children as well as a research tool to better understand how systems operate. Given the current stress in schools and other agencies as they struggle to accommodate increasing numbers of seriously disturbed children, it is most timely to review the methodology of Redl style consultation.

A special NIMH grant was awarded to Fritz Redl and Ruth Newman to study school consultation as a potential therapeutic and educational tool. Colleagues Howard Kitchner, MSW, and Claire Bloomberg, Master Teacher, were added to the team to enable participation in a range of settings from preschool through high school. Newman and Redl served as participants and supervisors of the project. The five public school settings, all in the District of Columbia, included two regular elementary schools, one special elementary, a large junior high and one senior high. The preschool was a cooperative. Such an array allowed age, setting and consulting process differential nuances to be analyzed. Acceptance by the system was contingent upon the understanding we were there to learn and were not to be in the way — an example of Redl's dicta that meaning well or being cast in the role of helper does not necessarily result in good works. The choice was to go where the conditions were most demanding to explore the potential of new practices.

The few consultation examples given here are from the final report, *Psychological Consultation in the Schools: A catalyst for learning* (Newman 1967). This project is an example of Redl's mode of clinical research.

The consultation style evolved directly from Redl's teaching and philosophy. While the particular system was demonstrated in schools, the concepts are generic as pertinent to other child serving institutions as to schools. The approach is as relevant to those who invite consultants as to those are invited as well as supervision within a system.

We cut through the many layers of theory written about consultation and went directly to the heart of the matter. Individual psychological dynamics and the power of ecological forces are combined. The focus is on problem solving. Such action oriented consultation means engagement and is a far cry from the artificial constraints imposed by typical consultation models. The goal is to become recognized as a part of the system.

Our first example illustrates the attention given to system factors which condition consultation. Rather than coming into a setting and doing the consultant's thing, it is a matter of assessing the ecological system and figuring out how service might best be rendered. Even though the immediate attention might be on a particular crisis deeper problems are recognized.

> The junior high presents some specific problems in consultation. For one thing, the junior high finds itself in charge of a greater variety and range of pupils than does the senior high. There are, for instance, a large number of youngsters who can barely, if at all, achieve graduation from the ninth grade and are simply serving time until they are sixteen. There are the

college-bound gifted students and the college-bound pedestrian pupils. There are the non-academic-minded youngsters who need a different kind of curriculum. There are the great majority of kids who are drifters and don't yet know what they want or what they are capable of. They are waiting until some life goal hits them, and if one is not allowed to have doubts about life goals at this age, we are living in a sad society. Adolescence blooms in its variegated form all over the junior high. Underdeveloped little youngsters who look like fifth-graders sit by the side of giants replete with bosoms or beards. There are the ones who already date and the ones who have entered into the phase of rebellion against adults — 'I won't' behavior, dress fashions, or out-and-out rudeness. There are those who have become adolescent isolates along with the pre-puberty friendly kids. Moreover, changes occur from day to day so that what one says of John or Sue in February may be meaningless in May. Considering the tremendous turmoil and challenge this age group presents, it is not difficult to see that staff problems run high, and one defense against problems one doesn't understand or feels helpless to deal with is denial.

Many junior high school teachers feel they are not good enough or experienced enough to make senior high school, which is considered a higher-status job. They have not been trained even as much as elementary-school teachers in the dynamics of growth and behavior. They are often at a loss to deal with the multitude of problems present and take refuge in concentrating on subject matter. Behavior problems are sent to detention hall or the assistant principal's office and seldom followed up by the teacher who sends, or the disciplinarian who receives. Rarely does one teacher get to know how a troubled or troublesome child behaves in his other courses, unless the child gets into so much trouble that he becomes a school scandal, or unless a consultant can institute staff meetings on a given case or a series of problems. Many a junior-high-school teacher feels that to stay on in junior high is a sign of low status, low success, and low recognition. Most of those who can, move up to the senior high, thus creating rapid staff turnover. This further fragments a junior-high student's learning experience by reducing the opportunities for stable teacher relationships. The difficulties and potentials of this age group require the best planning, understanding, and teaching. Many of those teachers who stay on feel like failures and act accordingly. Though there are many excellent teachers in the junior high, there are not enough and the low regard in which they are held discourages their staying there.

Consultation to the junior high, therefore, tends to concentrate on building up professional self-awareness and self-esteem among staff, acknowledging the multiplicity of the tasks, and indicating the opportunity that exists to reach a variety of kids on a variety of levels. It has to try to make clear the meaning of individual differences in growth and how a given piece of behavior may fit into developmental patterns. It must demonstrate or imply that the patterns a teacher likes or dislikes in a child may, at this age, be set for good or may vanish according to the response of the adult. Particularly important for the consultant in the junior high is the task, similar to that in the senior high, of setting up lines of communication among staff and among outside specialists: the psychological services of the school and the community, the clinics, the hospitals, and the vocational and recreational groups. Moreover, the school needs consultative help in receiving information, and using it, from the elementary schools, and in relaying appropriate, well-thought-out information to the senior high or vocational school. (Pp. 106-108)

Before any real work can be done, trust must be established, especially important when consultation is provided administrators and groups of pupils as well as teachers. For example, after some polite avoidance talk, the consultant was asked just what he was doing here, suspecting that he was going to add burdens. There was also anxiety that teachers were going to be "treated," or that they would have to keep extensive records. When the teacher's fears and questions were allayed, a remarkable increase in requests for consultation followed.

I had noticed earlier that the teacher and the children in Miss Z.'s classroom were unbearably tense. Miss Z. spent much time trying to out-yell the children, and she seemed too demanding and hostile toward them. Yet one had the impression that she wasn't this way most of the time. She had talked about the problem of yelling at the children and had asked me to suggest other ways of getting their attention which wouldn't be so wearing — and incidentally would not make her feel so bad.

In each of the conferences with Miss Z. she had two or three particular laments, usually about the most aggressive, demanding, or hostile children. Later the laments shifted to her feelings of futility about ever getting anywhere with some of her low-I.Q. or disturbed pupils. Still later, she was distressed by the frequent turnover of children in her class: She felt burdened by having to constantly regroup the class and handle the new pupils individually.

Her first concern was Jack, a big thirteen-year-old slow learner who seemed headed toward delinquency. He was often defiant and provocative with her, although she was not at all afraid of him physically. After listing his misdeeds, Miss Z. began to speculate about how this boy might feel about being in her class, which was sometimes referred to by the children as the "dumb class." She said that when he was transferred from a sixth-grade class he showed considerable embarrassment about being seen with this group, which contained several younger children. He would frequently line up with his old group in entering the building. She admitted that she had reached such a point of irritation with anything he did that she could no longer be objective about evaluating his behavior. I started her talking about another big boy in her room with whom she got along very well, and then she began to see that if this boy were doing some of the same things that Jack did she would not react so strongly. She agreed that she might try to use this second boy as a guide to controlling her overreactions to Jack, and she later reported that this seemed to work for her.

Later her concern was focused on a particularly difficult big girl who tended to try to control the class and was defiant and boisterous. After two or three meetings in which we discussed this child, Miss Z. raised the question of the necessity for her remaining in the special class. The girl had progressed to low performance for her regular grade level except in one subject. Within a few weeks we arranged to have her transferred back to her regular group, while she continued with Miss Z. for the one subject in which she needed individualized help.

It is noteworthy that week after week Miss Z. could raise meaningful issues to discuss with me and usually some plan could be worked out for the specific difficulties. However, she would periodically revert to a general complaint about the exasperations she experienced in trying to resolve permanently some of the problems in her special classroom. I began to raise with her what seemed to be the more basic issue she had to resolve: Since many of her chronic laments were inherent in the nature of teaching such special classes perhaps she had to think about whether this was the kind of teaching she wanted to continue to do.

Miss Z. gained some support from my comments about the similarity of her problems to those I had heard from special teachers in others schools. She could then begin to sort out specific problems about grouping, promotions, and so forth: When she could raise these questions with me, Miss Z. found she could formulate her views more clearly and thus make more productive use of conferences with her principal in which such issues could be resolved.

Aside from the help on specific issues which this teacher raised, the teacher appreciated the consultant's attention to her class. Such special classes in a regular school are often the forsaken classes. The teacher was supported by the fact that the consultant and principal had demonstrated that her situation warranted special attention. Thus her role was regarded seriously and her status enhanced. The principal was somewhat relieved because the teacher could begin to raise specific issues with which the principal could more easily help her. (Pp. 58-60)

Much of the consultation was done in groups—teacher pupil groups and volunteer parent groups. This next example traces the evolution of a pupil group, starting with one pupil in crisis which was converted into a positive group force. Consultants were often called upon to help when there was a serious crisis with a pupil. Fred has upset the system and especially the persons in charge by producing a mimeographed document about 'bad things' at the school. He has refused to talk and is about to be excluded. The stinging part of Fred's list was that most items had a basis in fact. Other students had pulled the fire alarm creating a great uproar as they walked out in Fred's support. The consultant used a Life Space Interview to bring down the escalation around Fred and then asked for a meeting with the "rebels" and in the process the Summit Group was formed.

I now come to one of the most interesting groups of kids I have ever worked with. It all began because of a widespread school crisis initiated by my old friend Fred. I was called to come to the school on urgent but unexplained business, asking if I would help out in a very bad situation. I asked if I could see all the students involved — some were members of the student government — and said I wanted to see if we could tackle some of the problems mentioned in the paper. There were four boys and six girls, and all of the tracks, from Honors to Basic, were represented. At first one teacher and I were the only interested, participating adults; later several teachers became actively involved. The group met every week for the rest of the school year and then continued on a monthly basis, with replacements made as members graduated. (It is still going on.) Within three weeks they were called "The Summit Group" and considered themselves a policy-planning group and did, indeed, affect the school and its policies.

We began by sorting out the problems Fred had brought up — which ones we, as a group within the school, could do anything about and which required more community social action. In time, members of the Summit Group became quite active in writing letters to the newspapers and making appearances on radio and television on subjects relevant to the city's problems or youth viewpoints.

The most immediate problem at Urban was the student body's fear of "outsiders" who broke into the building — often with knives, sometimes with guns — and made serious trouble. Groups of these outsiders, many of whom were dropouts from this and other nearby schools or unemployed graduates, hung around outside the building intimidating, blackmailing, and beating up Urban students on their way to and from school. The Summit Group made suggestions about what the students themselves could do and asked for faculty help in guarding doors. They also asked the adults to approach the police for better, and more understanding, coverage of the block at certain times, and this was the beginning of some work with the police on their attitudes toward and relations with teen-agers.

I suggested a weekly newsletter which could be cheaply mimeographed and distributed and would be quite distinct from the "ideal" school newspaper. Many of the teachers became interested and cooperative. English teachers, typing teachers, the faculty sponsor of student government, all helped and some worked hard on the actual physical production — proofreading, typing, mimeographing, collating, stapling. The newsletter came out for two cents a copy and became a regular feature of the school life. It served as a place for editorial comment on problems, for communication of school and personal events, for reports on programs, and for discussion of issues.

Another in-school problem that was tackled was the almost unbearable noise and confusion of the cafeteria. The Summit Group planned movies and social activities, record and combo playing at certain times during the lunch break. Cooperative teachers helped them to tempt masses of students out of the cafeteria and into fun activities away from the overcrowded lunchrooms and neighboring halls.

Of course there were issues that did not lend themselves to direct practical solutions, but these were, at least, aired and discussed. Child labor laws (originally made for their protection) prevented many youngsters from getting needed jobs after school.

As the year progressed the students trusted me with their fears and resentments, knowing I was not there to judge them and was genuinely interested in their feelings and ideas. Many faculty members cooperated in helping them with Summit Group projects. Beginning with the newsletter, and continuing on through the next year, the faculty sponsor of student government attended all their meetings. (Pp. 147-151)

There are many and diverse aspects to the Newman-Redl paradigm for open, action-oriented consultation. Often conversations were in informal settings, the teacher's lounge or lunch room: One hard to reach administrator much given to denial only felt free to talk when out for lunch. A series of seminars was requested to train teachers in teacher-parent collaboration. Direct confrontation was occasionally necessary: Consultants had to take risks to focus attention on certain problems and at the same time not be "used" by members of the system. First aid was administered to symptomatic crises but the basic process was to look for long term preventive interventions. A high school big brother program was developed for distraught elementary boys. A disastrous hiring and firing of an incredibly ill-suited teacher was worked through because of what his presence meant for teachers and the students. Teachers were brought to examine their prejudices and too low expectations for some students. The roots of their attitudes were explored. Separation anxiety of children was explored. Referral of individual cases was followed by requests for observation of the class as a whole, and discussion of professional competency usually followed. There was an instance where the staff were desperate, asking themselves how to contain an extremely disturbed, acting out pupil. An examination of the options led to seeking alternative care.

What are the principles which undergird Newman-Redl consultation?

1. There is flexibility of procedures but not of basic concepts. The unique nature of each setting and each situation determines the appropriate procedures.

2. The problem solving approach is based upon understanding individual and group dynamics as well as ecological forces.

3. Interact with all hierarchy levels in a system, from top administrator to pupil. Respect ecological forces and affective states of individuals whether or not they are self-acknowledged.

4. Effective consultation anticipates involvement in the nitty-gritty everyday life of the system. A consultant expects to be tested.

5. The presenting problem is often not the real problem, but one starts work there. Be willing to risk failure. Consultants are not magicians and usually a wide variety of services must be introduced to meet a system's needs.

6. Realistically take into account things as they are without being resigned to them; at the same time be aware of what should be changed. When changes do occur in one part of the system, anticipate that these may well cause new stresses in other parts of the system. Consultation on cases and putting out fires must be balanced with attention to underlying system issues.

7. Education and therapy are inexorably intertwined processes in the production of change.

REFERENCE

Newman, R.G. (1967) *Psychological consultation in the schools: a catalyst for learning*. New York: Basic Books.

I Wonder What Fritz Would Say?

Thom Garfat, PhD

Director of Treatment
Youth Horizons

EDITOR'S NOTE: We begin with Nicholson's tribute to Redl stemming from the excitement of a young worker 'finding Fritz.' Garfat uses a dramatic format to remind us that this can still happen if new professionals are introduced to Redl's work. Those who live with children will respond to his vivid images and living snapshots which provide penetrating answers beyond the superficial advice common in current training. Redl had an abiding interest in professionalizing the 'living with' on the line workers: Garfat shows how residential treatment would benefit by taking Redl to heart.

Well, today's my first day. Sometimes I thought it would never come. It seemed to take forever to get here but, here I am. God, I hope I do okay. I've wanted to be a Child Care Worker for years, almost forever it seems to me when I look back on it all. Not that it took a long time, like a doctor or anything like that, but still . . . four years to get my Bachelors degree, all those hours in practicuums, all those classes, exams, summer jobs and starving winters. Seems like it took forever. But here I am. First job, first day, first shift. God, I hope I do okay. I hope I remember all the stuff I learned: especially the stuff by that guy Redl. Practical stuff . . . it made a lot of sense compared to some of the other authors I had to read. I wonder if the other child care workers here have read his stuff. I guess they must have. Surely everybody's read it. I better be careful

---

about what I say. I don't want to look like one of those 'fresh out of school know-it-alls.' Maybe I'll just keep my mouth shut for a while and see how it goes.

Well, here I am. May as well go in. I wonder what these kids will be like. What was it that Redl said . . . (Redl & Wineman 1952)

> They are the children who cannot meet the challenge of the tasks of every day life without becoming a helpless bundle of drives. (p. 15)

Not a lot of information to go on but probably as good as anything else I ever read. There was more to it than that, but that's good enough for now. But I would like to know their classification: that would at least help me know how to approach them.

> Will you please just forget about diagnosis? (1982, p. 4)

I go up the stairs and open the door. I hope that the kids will like me. I want to get along with them, I think it's so important but like Redl said they "can't like you too much because you set the rules" (op. cit. p. 7).

I step inside and look around for the office. A doorway stands open in the corridor and I head for it thinking that must be it. It is. I peer inside. No one's there. Logs and files lie on the desk. I wonder why it's open. Perhaps it's one of the ways they demonstrate their trust of the children. I remember learning that's important, but Redl has something to say about that as well . . . (op. cit.)

> . . . Adults must definitely know what kinds of things and situations expose these youngsters to uncontrollable temptation and should not expose them to more of it than their ego can be expected to cope with at that time. (p. 47)

I wonder where the staff is. I'd like to know if the open office with everything 'exposed' says more about the kids or the staff. I remember the rest of that paragraph where Redl (op. cit.) says that it is our job to "support what ego strength has remained, not to undermine it by exposing it to entirely unmanageable strain"

(p. 47). I close the door as I leave the office just in case. I decide to wander around the house to see if I can find anyone.

At first, it seems too messy to me. In the living room someone has forgotten to put away some games lying on the floor and I stack them neatly on the coffee table as I pass. I pick up a few glasses and some orange peels and head off in search of the kitchen. The pictures in the corridor are hanging crooked and as I straighten them I notice that the frames could use washing. The kitchen is no better than the rest of the house. "God," I think, "doesn't this place have a housekeeper? Doesn't anyone make these kids clean up the place?" I wonder to myself what Redl would have to say (op. cit.).

> Adults in a treatment home need the ability to sacrifice what personal style of housekeeping they happen to be most enamored with to the clinical strategy needed at a certain time. (p. 48)

Well, I guess if I'm going to listen to Redl and what he had to say, my reaction says more about me that anything else. But it is hard to set your own values aside even if Redl says you should. I guess that's why we spent time on self-awareness in our classes last year. After all, I'm here to deal with their business, not mine.

I don't find anyone in the kitchen so I decide to take a further stroll through the house to see what I can find and get a feel for the place. Maybe it will tell me more about the program or the kids who live here. I don't know much about them except that they are pre-adolescents.

It seems like a pretty average place. Parts of the house could use some paint and there's surely nothing fancy about it. I guess Redl would approve. I remember reading (op. cit.) that he thought that it was important that the environment not be too unfamiliar or different from the child's natural environment so as to avoid "sociological shock" and the "newness panic" that could come about if the environment was too much of a change for the child to adjust to easily (p. 43).

I see that the furniture is sturdy stuff, the kind that can take a little rough and tumble, or the occasional outburst, without coming apart at the seams. Most of it looks like it's been around for a while and has seen a number of kids pass through. But it's not worn to the point of looking like somebody else's discard. It has a healthy, lived-in, inviting kind of look to it. It feels like the kind of place where you're supposed to be comfortable. I'm sure he'd approve of that too. He (op. cit.) had a lot to say about the environment, and the tools available in working with kids (43-45; 192-198).

But I better go and find the staff. If I don't find them soon they'll think I was late.

I wander through other parts of the house looking here and there; 'scoping the territory' as the kids in that last place used to say. Finally I hear sounds — laughter, shouting and playful cries — and they lead me to the backyard. From the porch I see two or three youngsters throwing a ball and two others sitting at a picnic table playing cards. Off to the side I see a young woman talking to two youngsters who look about ready to kill each other. Another staff, also female, sits under the tree consoling a young girl of about ten years. I can tell by how the staff is sitting that she's keeping an eye on all the action over the child's shoulder. She catches my attention and signals me to come over.

As I approach the little girl runs off to join the others at the table and I stammer an apology to Carol, the Child Care Worker, "Sorry, Carol, I didn't mean to frighten her away."

"Don't worry," she replies with a slight twinkle showing in her eyes. "Nancy was just getting a little 'tax-free love and affection' (op. cit. p. 61) and she'd taken just about all she could allow herself to take for the moment. She was looking for a good excuse to leave without having to get angry and if you hadn't come along I would have had to ease her into something else. That's a hurdle she hasn't learned to get over on her own yet and I could sense the anxiety building up (op. cit. p.175-78). Once you get to know Nancy, you'll sense it yourself but like all the kids, she expresses her anxiety in her own unique way." She paused for a minute as if asking herself a question. "I think you and I should go in the kitchen for a few minutes and talk. I'll just take a second to set it up and then we can go."

Carol stood up and signaling to her partner, who by now had drifted back into the ball game with her two young charges, she let everyone know that she was going to be in the kitchen with me.

Then, after introducing me to all the children and her co-worker Sally she led me to the kitchen. We sat by the window, overlooking the yard, close to the open door. When all the kids saw her settled in the window, they returned to their play and she turned to me.

"So, what do you think of our house?"

"What I've seen I like a lot. Of course I haven't been all the way through but there seems to be a lot of space and it has a homey lived-in kind of look. It feels comfortable," I responded, not sure where she was going with this.

She knew. "I'm glad you noticed the space. It's really important to us. Like Fritz said, "space can be of the utmost importance" (op. cit. p. 45).

"Fritz who?"

She laughed again; I realized that it was friendly so it didn't offend me. "Why, Redl, or course. You do know his work, don't you?"

"Well, well, sure," I stammered. "We studied it in class."

"Good. You see, around here we're really committed to his ideas and approaches. None of us think that he has all the answers for all of the kids we see, but in terms of understanding how to work with these kids no one else has provided such a good foundation for programming." She paused for a moment as she surveyed the scene in the yard smiling and recognizing the kids who caught her eye. "What do you think of his work?"

"As you know, I'm pretty new to all of this and I haven't read as much as you but I do remember when I read *Children Who Hate* (Redl & Wineman 1951). For the first time I felt like I was understanding how children come to be troubled. And when I read the chapter on 'The Delinquent Ego and It's Techniques,' especially the section on being a 'friend without influence,' I understood the difference between the relationship as a goal and the relationship as a tool in working with kids. It helped me to understand how children can really like a staff without the staff being able to influence them" (op. cit. p. 224).

"Oh, me too! I remember that I had been working in the field for a number of years before I read that," Carol responded. "As I read that book, so much of my experience seemed to make more sense. That was about ten years ago and I remember thinking that it could have been written only yesterday. I heard somebody say that once and thought at the time that it's so true. That book is as useful and meaningful today as when Fritz and David Wineman wrote it in 1951 (Garfat 1987).''

I was curious and had to ask. "You always refer to him as Fritz. Did you know him? Was he a friend?"

Again the light laugh as she kept her eye on the yard. For a moment she and her co-worker exchanged glances and Sally signaled to her that everything was fine. "No, I didn't know him. But we all feel as if we did. His work is so intimately familiar to all of us that I feel as if he was my personal teacher. It's something about the way that he writes . . . as if he's talking directly to you. As if he is a friend.''

She paused for a minute. "I did hear him talk though, once at a Child Care Conference. I remember watching this little man, with an accent so strong that I could hardly understand him, saying some of the most practical things I ever heard about working with troubled kids; and by then I'd been in the field for years. It was right after that that I read all his stuff and realized that the school I went to had cheated us all by not teaching his work. I'm glad to see that they do now.''

"I know what you mean," I responded. "I read all the other things on the class list but nothing else was as personal or useful as his work. For somebody new to the field it's as if he takes you by the hand and says 'this is what a good program should look like; this is what it should feel like; this is how the children should experience it.' When I read *Controls From Within* (Redl & Wineman 1952), I wondered why there wasn't more writing like it in the field.''

"Because there's only been one Fritz," Carol replied over her shoulder as she moved outside to redirect a couple of kids whose discussion was getting heated up. She was back in a minute and the children who were about to fight were laughing. "As Fritz points out,'' she said, "a little humour at the right moment can really help.''

"But like he also said," I replied, "we shouldn't assume that 'any tense or difficult situation could be successfully handled by humorous reaction' (op. cit. p. 75). That's something else I appreciate about his work, he always cautioned against over-generalizing." I was glad that I knew his work as well as I did, but I'd never realized how enjoyable it could be to discuss it with someone who practiced it.

"That's true," Carol came back, "when, how, for how long, by whom, where. All of these were important to him. Like when he talked about timing; as in how long a consequence should last for."

"I remember when we discussed that in class," I responded. "That's a hot issue even today. Like how long should a kid be sent to his room for: five minutes? ten? half an hour? But I can't remember what Redl had to say about it."

"Well then," Carol said, the laugh coming up again, "let that be your first task of the day. Go into the office and get the copy of *Controls From Within*, and read pages 116 to 119. When you're finished come find me and we'll continue."

With that Carol got up and went back outside. I headed back to the office. Above the desk, which was facing the wall, I found a well-worn copy of the book and sat down to read.

Like always, I found the language to be clear and the ideas useful and well-demonstrated through a little vignette. One line still stays with me even today (Redl & Wineman 1952): "The development of skills in clinically adequate timing constitutes one of the most important problems of the training and self-training of staff" (p. 118).

I wish we'd spent more time on that in the class. A note penciled in the margin referred me to another article (Redl 1982) where I found a more specific reference to our conversation. A line from that article stays with me as well: ". . . longer does not mean that effects are achieved faster" (Pp. 5-6).

I sat in the chair and thought about what I had read for a few minutes. Redl's writings will do that: make you think. I went out to find Carol and Sally.

I passed Sally in the kitchen doing a "Guilt Squeeze" (Redl & Wineman 1951, p. 257-260) with one of the youngsters she had been with when I arrived. She didn't turn from the child as I passed and I remember how Redl had talked about the need to attend to the children when you're interviewing them. Carol was in the living room with a small group debriefing the afternoon. I sat down and joined her. Her work was true to everything Redl had to say about group interviews being able to serve "the same clinical goals and

functions as individual interviewing." I could see where I was going to have to review his writings on interviews and interviewing
techniques if I was going to work here. (Redl & Wineman 1952,
p. 246-273)

When the group was over and it was time to move into the dining
room to eat, Carol caught me for a quick aside. "Did you read the
article on timing and the discussion about longer and faster?"

"I did," I replied. "It made me think."

"Good," she said, "Making people think is probably what Fritz
did best. It may have been his major contribution to the field. Not
what he said, but how it makes you think: like his comments on
what we mean by the use of the word 'therapeutic' (1966, pp. 72-
29). The more we think about what we do, the better we serve the
children. And I'm sure Fritz would agree that that's why we're
here."

I thought for another minute as we seated ourselves at the table
and then said to Carol, "I think I'll call him Fritz too."

"That's good," Carol laughed. "But let me tell you a little technique I learned from Sally. Whenever I look at a situation, or run
into something I'm not sure about and I don't really know what to
think or do, I ask myself a question and it helps me every time."

"What's the question?" I asked, anxious to learn.

"I wonder what Fritz would say?" she laughed.

REFERENCES

Garfat, T. (1987). Words that have meaning. *Residential Treatment for Children and Youth*, *5*(2), pp 5-12.

Redl, F. & Wineman, D. (1951). *Children Who Hate*. New York: The Free Press.

Redl, F. & Wineman, D. (1952). *Controls From Within: Techniques for the Treatment of the Aggressive Child*. New York: The Free Press.

Redl, F. (1966). *When We Deal with Children: Selected Writings*. New York: The Free Press.

Redl, F. (1982). Child Care Work, *Journal of Child Care*, *1*(2), 3-9.

A Brief Orientation to Redl's Writing

William C. Morse, PhD

University of Michigan
University of South Florida

Garfat has just illustrated how Redl is a sourcebook for those who deal directly with distraught children hours on end. In addition to realistic handling advice, Redl also quickens the insight and theoretical sophistication of the highly experienced. Because of his agility in moving from indelible example to underlying psychological concept, Redl speaks to all professionals who work with disturbed children.

The present special issue whets the appetite to read (or reread) original Redl. There is no concordance or even complete bibliography of his work. The suggestions which follow are only a few of those the editor has found useful in practice and in staff development.

For those interested in residential therapy, two major joint works are most rewarding:

> Redl, F. & Wineman, D. (1951), *Children Who Hate*. New York: Free Press.
> Redl, F. & Wineman, D. (1952). *Controls from Within: Techniques for the Treatment of The Aggressive Child*. New York: Free Press.

Redl's articles have appeared in German and English in a wide variety of Journals from *Parents* to the *American Journal of Orthopsychiatry*. Since he never wrote down to a readership, they are all valuable. Fortunately many of his writings have been collected in one volume which also contains the most complete bibliography we have covering the years 1931 to 1965.

Redl, F. (1966) *When We Deal With Children*. New York: Free Press.

In this collection, he somewhat revised and provided an explanatory introduction for each reprint. While additional articles can be found by searching his bibliography, the following suggestions come from his book and the pages refer to that volume.

Redl was insistent that practice be related to developmental psychology and he probed the psychology of both of pre-adolescence and adolescence.

Pre Adolescents: "What Makes Them 'Tic'?" Pp. 395-409.
The Concept of Ego Disturbance and Ego Support. Pgs. 125-147.
What Do We Do About the "Facts of Life." Pp. 378-385.
Psychoanalysis and Education. Pp. 147-151.
Discipline in Classroom Practice. Pp. 254-308.

An overarching concern of Redl was of course milieu treatment:

The Concept of a "Therapeutic Milieu." Pp. 68-94.
Framework for Our Discussions on Punishment. Pp. 355-377.
How Do I Know When I Should Stop It? Pp. 346-349.
This Time We Should Not Interfere — But Why? Pp. 349-354.
The Life Space Interview — Strategy And Techniques. Pp. 35-67.
Improvement Panic and Improvement Shock. Pp. 95-124.

Of course we know Redl as the one who has so much to teach about groups:

The Art of Group Composition. Pp. 236-253.
Group Emotion and Leadership. Pp. 155-196.
Resistance in Therapy Groups. Pp. 214-223.
The Phenomena of Contagion and "Shock Effect." Pp. 197-213.

Finally, his insights on delinquent behavior could change our understanding of delinquency and what we can do about it:

Who Is Delinquent. Pp. 418-426.
The Virtues of Delinquent Children. Pp. 461-466.
The Psychology of Gang Formation and the Treatment of Juvenile Delinquents. Pp. 224-235.

Printed and bound by CPI Group (UK) Ltd, Croydon, CR0 4YY

22/10/2024

01777620-0006